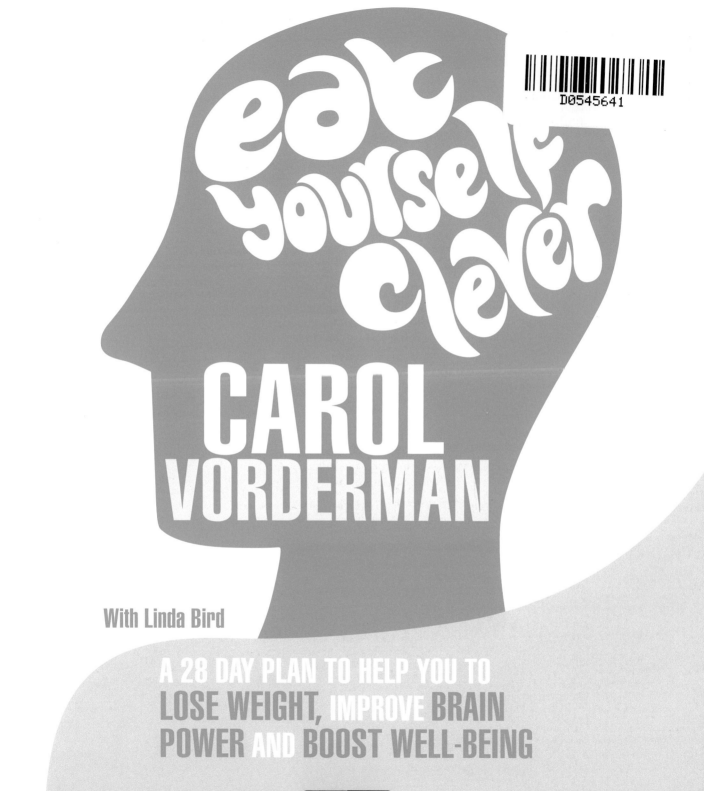

eat yourself clever

CAROL VORDERMAN

With Linda Bird

A 28 DAY PLAN TO HELP YOU TO
LOSE WEIGHT, IMPROVE BRAIN
POWER AND BOOST WELL-BEING

Virgin BOOKS

D0545641

Acknowledgements
With thanks to Anita Bean for all her guidance and expertise, and Elisabeth Wilson for her additional research. Thanks also to Lizzie Harris for her inspiring recipes.

While the authors have made every effort to ensure that the information in this book is as accurate and up-to-date as possible, it is advisory only and should not be used as an alternative to seeking specialist medical advice. The authors and publisher cannot be held responsible for actions that may be taken by a reader as a result of reliance on the information contained in this book, which are taken entirely at the reader's own risk.

First published in Great Britain in 2008 by
Virgin Books Ltd
Thames Wharf Studios
Rainville Road
London
W6 9HA

A catalogue record for this book is available from the British Library.

ISBN 978 0 7535 1355 2

The paper used in this book is a natural, recyclable product made from wood grown in sustainable forests. The manufacturing process conforms to the regulations of the country of origin.

Art direction by Dan Newman

Printed and bound in Germany

Picture credits: Pages 4, 7, 16, 22, 29, 35, 37, 39, 55, 56, 58, 62, 65, 91, 94, 111, 115, 124 and 137 © Karl Grant. All other images © Shutterstock

Contents

Introduction

It happens to the best of us.

We all have those days when we find we're just not as mentally efficient as we'd like to be … Perhaps we can't seem to concentrate on the task in hand, or find it harder to remember names and numbers, or where we left the car keys (or the car itself!). Or perhaps we can't access that word or phrase that's on the tip of our tongue, or do calculations in our head as quickly as we used to.

It's true that cognitive decline is part of the ageing process, and that over time our mental faculties will start to diminish. That's a fact of life.

Unfortunately, in this culture of anti-ageing, where people will willingly go under the knife to knock a decade or so off their face, it's not so easy to surgically enhance the brain.

The fast-moving, stressful world we live in doesn't help our moments of brain-drain. In fact, in many ways it's responsible for it. Our lives are stressful, we're working long hours and are often skimping on sleep, which plays havoc with our powers of concentration and retention.

We're bombarded with information, flashing screens, and are fed all sorts of chemical substances in our food, so it's little wonder our faculties and senses aren't always as sharp as they perhaps should be.

Mood also plays a role. When we're stressed, down or anxious our brain's chemistry is altered and our reactions or ability to digest and act on information are impaired.

Add to this the constant pressures on women in particular to conform to a physical ideal (slim, pert, perfect) – and the fact that as a result many young women starve or malnourish themselves to attain that ideal, and you can see how easy it is for our brains to lack important nutrients.

So what can we do to slow down cognitive decline? How can we ensure that our brain is functioning at its best possible level, whatever our age? And what kind of anti-ageing tools are there to help preserve our memory?

The answer is nutrition.

The good news is that growing scientific evidence suggests that diet may play an important role in improving the way your mind works. Eating the right types of foods and cutting the junk provide the mind with the nutrients it needs for optimal function and can result in a dramatic improvement in your health, mental performance and mood.

Think about it. You go to work without breakfast and by mid-morning you're hungry and fantasising about bacon sandwiches or chocolate biscuits. Your brain, having been made to fast for hours since suppertime, is short on the essential nutrients it needs to function optimally. Little wonder you can't make head or tail of that tricky work project.

Perhaps you're a slave to the latest diet fad – hoping that by cutting out carbs, or living off grapefruit or cabbage soup, you can finally shed those stubborn pounds. But being preoccupied with food – and weight – and bingeing or starving as a result are further impediments to a fully functioning sharp mind.

Now's the time to forget about brawn and focus on brain. The best news of all is that what's good for the brain is going to do wonders for your body too. By eating the right food to get your brain in gear chances are you'll shed pounds, shape up and notice a big improvement in your moods too. It could be a win-win situation.

So how does it work?

The book has been designed to help you understand how the brain works, get a grip on your eating habits, lose weight, improve your brain power and help wellbeing.

It's based on the premise that good nutrition helps improve your brain power (and there are plenty of studies that confirm this) and that a healthy diet full of the right kinds of foods also improves concentration, mood, learning ability and memory, slowing the decline in brain function that occurs with age.

Chapter by chapter we'll explore how the brain works – what it needs to function, and which kinds of food provide the best nourishment. We'll look at specific foods that help boost mood and which ones have a knock-on effect on brain function. We'll also investigate the cause of the dreaded cravings – how they can scupper a diet, and your brain power – and what you can do to control them once and for all.

There's also a section on which bad habits to avoid – smoking, high levels of alcohol, sugar – and how to find out what they're doing to your poor brain!

How can we ensure our brain is functioning at its best? The answer is nutrition

And for those ready to turn over a new leaf and make some brain-boosting resolutions, there's a section outlining some important good habits to adopt to help bring your brain up a notch or two – for example, getting more sleep, taking more exercise, finding time for relaxation can help both your waistline and your brain. (There are ways to make those resolutions easier to follow, too.)

The final chapter, the 28-Day Plan, is a day-by-day eating programme with delicious but simple recipes you can whip up for the whole family.

And weight loss? Think about it. By improving mood, happiness and the way you think you'll make better food choices and learn to control your weight without dieting. The food plan is inspiring, but not prescriptive, so you can mix and match days and recipes to suit your lifestyle and schedule.

The beauty of the programme is that there'll be a wonderful ripple effect, because, if the brain works better, you'll feel better emotionally, and you may lose unwanted pounds.

In fact, once you start choosing the foods that can best benefit your brain, the whole family benefits. Children can improve learning (and behaviour) and adults may slow or stop the age-related deterioration in memory and concentration.

Try it and see. And who knows, in 28 days, you may find you'll just sail through that crossword or sudoku (or even find your car!).

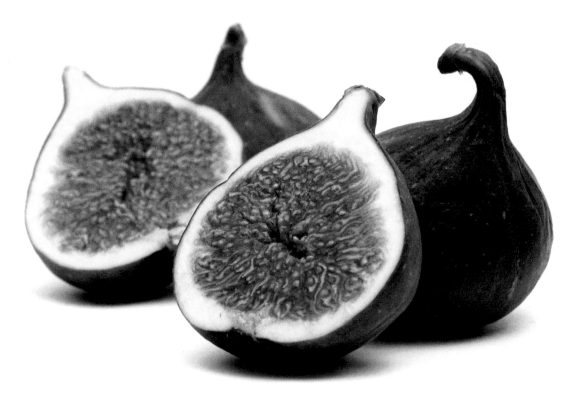

Chapter 1
Brain Power
Food for thought

Ever skipped breakfast and spent the morning feeling hungry and unable to concentrate, or felt drowsy and mentally sluggish after a big meal? Have you snacked on sugary biscuits or chocolate and felt an immediate energy burst, only be left feeling tired, drained and emotionally low soon after? Or felt a strong craving for a certain food when you were stressed or feeling down?

The relationship between what we eat and our mental state is a powerful and complex one. The examples above are probably some of the most common ways in which food affects how we think and feel, and I'm sure you've experienced one if not all of them at some point.

But, as well as making us feel a certain way, the food we eat can also have an effect on our mental ability – in short, it is possible to eat yourself cleverer.

The food we eat can have a significant effect on our brains. What we consume every day can influence our mood and behaviour; it can alter how we think and react; it can even affect our ability to concentrate.

Not only that, but research suggests that food and diet may have played a role in the development of the human brain and intelligence over time. Scientists have discovered that certain populations of early man, which appear to have been more intelligent than others, congregated around the coasts. They would have gathered seafood – known to be rich in essential fatty acids necessary for brain growth.

So, it seems that, right from the dawn of mankind, what we eat has affected our brain power, and continues to do so today.

In the following chapters, you'll learn all about which foods contain the nutrients that can help boost your mental ability. You'll also discover what to avoid. But before we go into more detail about this, it's useful to know a little bit about how the brain works and the main foods you need to keep it operating at full capacity.

How does the brain 'work'?

Your brain consists of billions and billions of cells. Most of these are simple 'glial' cells – the 'glue' that holds the brain together. The glial cells are also responsible for supporting and nourishing the neurons – these cells carry electrical signals to each other and all over the body.

Each neuron is connected to up to 10,000 neighbouring neurons. The connections between them are made via axons and dendrites: axons carry signals away from the neuron, and dendrites to them. Between each axon and dendrite is a tiny gap, the synapse. Signals are passed across the synapse by the release of chemicals – the neurotransmitters.

It's useful to know a little about these neurotransmitters, because certain foods can stimulate and inhibit their release, which can have a powerful effect on how you're feeling.

The neurotransmitters

These are the brain chemicals that make everything possible.

- **Serotonin** – this 'feel-good' chemical has the ability to make us feel serene, happy and calm. It promotes contentment and sleep.
- **Dopamine** – responsible for 'get up and go' – it's the great arouser and motivator and important for assertiveness and sexual arousal. Dopamine is necessary for fine muscle coordination and those with Parkinson's disease have a diminished ability to synthesise it.
- **Noradrenaline** – like its brother adrenaline, noradrenaline livens you up. It's needed to stimulate brain activity and for concentration and for the formation of memories.
- **Acetylcholine** – is necessary for attention, learning and memory. A deficiency is directly related to impaired thinking ability.
- **Endorphins and Enkephalins** – like their relatives, the opiates, these make you feel happy and reduce stress. They also reduce pain.

Brain power …

Believing that you can become more intelligent can make it so. Studies from Columbia and Stanford Universities have shown that children who believed that they could 'grow' their intelligence, and that intelligence could be expanded, performed better academically than their peers. Explaining to children how they can improve their brain function and learning could do a lot to improve their future performance.

Eat Yourself Clever Carol Vorderman

Getting to know your brain

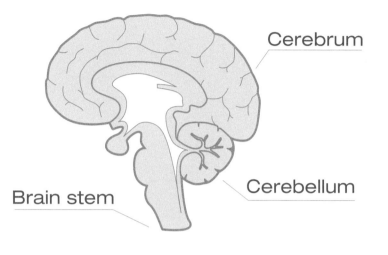

Cerebrum

Cerebellum

Brain stem

Brain stem

The brain stem is one of the oldest parts of the brain and controls many involuntary reactions such as breathing, digestion and heart rate.

Cerebellum

Lying at the back of the brain, tucked behind the brain stem, the cerebellum is known as 'the little brain'. The cerebellum is responsible for co-ordinating muscles, reflexes and maintaining balance.

Cerebrum

The cerebrum is the brain that we are most familiar with – the multi-grooved walnut-shaped organ. The cerebrum is covered by the cortex and neocortex, extra layers of 'grey' matter to facilitate sophisticated thinking. It is divided into two hemispheres which are mirrors of each other (the right and left hemispheres). Each hemisphere has four distinct parts: the frontal, parietal, temporal and occipital lobes. Each lobe processes the information coming from the opposite side of the body.

The frontal lobes: here is the part of the brain that primarily makes you 'you'. It is where you do your thinking and planning, where you decide how to respond to an urge coming from your unconscious brain – in other words, the home of your personality and morality.

The left hemisphere is the 'clever' side of the brain, which is responsible for speech, writing and calculation. It is where information is processed sequentially, so noises for example are recognised as distinct sounds.

The right hemisphere is the 'creative' side of the brain, where the parts recognised by the left hemisphere are 'seen' as a whole. It is the right-hand brain that perceives and constructs patterns from the information gathered by the left-hand brain.

left brain or right brain?

Which side of your brain predominates? Find out with our quiz. It's a bit of a fun and shouldn't be taken too seriously, but at the same time, it might give you some insight into how you respond to life's challenges and how to play to your strengths.

1) How often do you find yourself in those situations where you feel that you may be out of your depth?
a) Hardly ever. You hate that feeling and do what you can to prepare for contingencies.
b) Fairly often, every month or so at least. Probably more.

2) While you're on the phone do you tend to doodle in
a) words?
b) pictures?

3) When you're being given directions to a place you've never visited before do you prefer
a) instructions to use in conjunction with a map?
b) just the address? Instructions bore you to tears. You'll find it or you'll phone.

4) A colleague in your team has a good idea. You ask how he came up with it and he says 'just a hunch'. You react by
a) ordering in-depth research and analysis to see if the idea has worked anywhere else.
b) going with it. You intuitively feel he's right.

5) Describe your bedroom in one word. Is that word
a) a descriptive word describing colour or period furniture?
b) an emotional word describing the 'feel' of the room?

Mostly a)s
You are more likely to have a left-hand brain. You are logical, good at reasoning and with a terrific eye for detail. You are gifted with words both written and spoken and are valued for your persuasiveness and negotiation skills.

Mostly b)s
You are more likely to have a right-hand brain. You consider intuition as useful as your analytical abilities in reaching a decision. You get results; thinking creatively and flexibly, your 'out of the box' ideas are invaluable to yourself and others.

Eat Yourself Clever Carol Vorderman

Why keeping busy really does help mend a broken heart

The emotional right-hand side of the brain generates melancholy. When the left-hand side of the brain is 'quiet' (relatively unoccupied), it is easy for these right-hand side feelings to dominate. So by keeping busy – writing, planning, organising – actively utilising your left-hand brain, you inhibit the emotional response of the right-hand side.

The 'unconscious' mind

The limbic system is a very 'old' part of the brain and is responsible for actions relating to basic urges and emotions, and directs the behaviour that helps us survive. It consists of the thalamus, hypothalamus, amygdala and hippocampus. The thalamus allows greater processing of incoming information; the hypothalamus controls the internal environment of the body; the hippocampus is responsible for our long-term memory; and the amygdala is the part of the brain where fear is generated.

The addictive brain

Why can some of us never get enough, whether it's enough drinks, drugs, food or shoes?

Desires have their origin in the brain. Addictions are likely to prove more complicated than a simple matter of brain chemistry, but scientists have several theories as to why some of us are addicts. One of these is the 'reward deficiency syndrome'. Some of us (the addicts) have brains which, even when a desire is met, cannot switch off their appetites.

The 'reward', the feeling of satisfaction, is dependent on a rush of neurotransmitters but some people (as many as one in four) don't get that rush. These people keep consuming, desperate for the feeling of satiety, in an elusive attempt to experience 'enough'.

Limber up your limbic system

You can actively prime your limbic system to keep you happy. Smell travels straight to centres in the limbic system. Next time you're happy, sniff a favourite scent – lavender, rose oil or a favourite perfume – whatever you like. Then, repeat on a few more occasions. Very soon your limbic system will be primed and you can use that fragrance to soothe and calm you. You will have 'hardwired' your brain to associate it with happy times.

So how do desires get switched off?

Stimulus (such as hunger or the sight of an ice cream van)

↓

Limbic system
(unconscious urge)

↓

Cortex (conscious desire)

↓

Body (action to satisfy desire)

↓

Limbic system
(neurotransmitter such as dopamine released)

↓

Feeling of satisfaction.

Feeding your mind

What does your brain need to flourish? In the following pages we'll explore exactly what you need to eat (and what you must avoid) to have a brain that is operating at maximum capacity and that will stay healthy and productive. However, in short what your brain needs is an old-fashioned 'balanced diet'. So above all, your brain needs all three of the major nutrients to be healthy.

Fat

You will have read a great deal about how various different fats affect your weight and cardiovascular health. Less attention is given to the role of fat in keeping your brain healthy. But now doctors believe that fat is essential for regulating mood. On the other hand, too much saturated fat (from animal sources) leads to the same sort of artery clogging (atherosclerosis) that results in heart disease. If an artery in the brain is clogged in the same way, the result can be stroke or vascular dementia.

As with all fat, it is important to get enough of the good type and restrict the bad. Most of us who eat fish or meat each day, take milk in our tea or coffee, snack on yoghurt and enjoy the odd biscuit don't have to worry about getting enough fat.

But we can do a lot to improve brain function by actively choosing to eat healthy fats rather than unhealthy ones. These healthy fats are the omega-3 fatty acids found in fish and the mono-unsaturated and polyunsaturated fats found in olive oil and other healthy oils such as hemp and rape; nuts and seeds; avocadoes and olives. There is more on the unhealthy fats that you should avoid later on in this book.

Why we need the healthy fats:

- to form the brain's cells' (neuronal) membranes.
- to form the protective myelin sheath that allows faster communication (it is 70% fat).
- to protect us from depression. Deficiency in certain fats can make us more vulnerable to depression, according to research by the US's National Institutes of Health.
- to boost IQ. Fat builds brain power. The reason breast-fed infants score higher in IQ tests is thought to be that their mothers' milk transfers exactly the right ratio of the right fats.

Healthy swaps

Swap: sausages and other red meats for oily fish such as herring, mackerel and sardines
Swap: bread spread with butter for bread dunked into extra-virgin olive oil
Swap: crisps for olives
Swap: a couple of biscuits for a handful of nuts
Swap: jam on toast for sardines on toast

Protein

If fat makes up the brain cells, proteins allow messages to be sent between the neurons. Most neurotransmitters are made up of amino acids, which are the building blocks of proteins. We need to eat protein in order to ensure a steady supply of neurotransmitters.

This is one reason why what we eat can have such a profound effect on what we think and feel. If you eat a piece of fish for lunch, you are going to feel far more alert and productive in the afternoon than if you had eaten a bowl of pasta – that's partly because the fish will break down to the amino acid tyrosine, which promotes release of noradrenaline and dopamine. These neurotransmitters will keep you motivated and focused right through the so-called mid-afternoon slump.

You only need a couple of servings of protein a day to keep your brain working actively – but it's best to get them during the day, at breakfast and lunch, so they can get to work keeping your concentration high when you need it. Save a big bowl of pasta or plate of rice for supper.

Which proteins to eat
There are eight amino acids and dietary proteins are classified depending on how many they supply:

Complete proteins: these supply all eight of the amino acids and in-clude fish, meat, eggs, cheese, milk and yoghurt. You can see from this that a vegan (who excludes meat and dairy products) has to put a little more thought into his or her diet to ensure a healthy mix of proteins.

Incomplete proteins: foods such as grains, legumes, seeds and nuts provide some of the amino acids but not all of them. They need to be eaten in combination to form complete proteins – for instance, rice and beans together is a classic complete protein which millions around the world have depended on as a dietary staple.

Carbohydrates

Fats make up brain cells, protein 'fires' them off but it's carbohydrate which is needed to fuel them. Your brain runs on the carbohydrate glucose, and because neurons don't store it, they need a constant supply. Deprived of carbohydrate, your body will break down fat and muscle (protein) to get enough glucose but whereas carbohydrates 'burn clean', fat and protein leave harmful residues which your body has to process and eliminate.

It's not just that they break down to the food of choice. Carbohydrates also supply the amino acid tryptophan and this is necessary for production of serotonin, so essential to maintaining an even mood.

Interesting studies on rats show that a steady supply of glucose is needed if we want to concentrate and at the same time retain a good memory. It appears that during periods of intense concentration, glucose is drained away from the parts of the brain responsible for laying down memory. When rats are young they can just about cope with having to do two major brain functions at once, but as they age, memory slips as they try to maintain concentration. Scientists have speculated that the human brain may work the same way and recommend that getting enough carbohydrate is essential for maintaining brain function.

Another study showed that when the memories of older adults were assessed, they performed better having eaten carbohydrate foods within an hour of the tests. Carbohydrates give better memory performance than either protein or fat.

Carbohydrates for brain power

When you consider that your brain uses up about 25% of your calorie intake a day, it's clear that for effective brain power, you need to eat superior fuel every day. The best possible fuel is the type of carbohydrate foods – grains, legumes, fruits and vegetables – known as unrefined (or complex) carbohydrates that reach your body in their natural state, not messed around too much by factory processing. The unrefined carbohydrates are broken down relatively slowly by your body, ensuring a steady supply of energy to your brain.

On the other hand, the refined carbohydrates are those found in processed foods (such as biscuits, sugary drinks and sweets). The body breaks them down rapidly and a sudden surge of sugar hits your blood stream. This is the so-called 'sugar rush', which is just as quickly followed by a 'sugar crash', when the glucose is used up and you suddenly feel exhausted and irritable, 'running on empty'. And of course, that state is disastrous for your mental focus.

There is more on the adverse effects of the wrong sort of carbs later. The important thing is to remember to get enough of the right sort.

When it comes to helping us choose the healthiest carbohydrates, the GI (glycaemic index) is invaluable. Each foodstuff has a value dependent on the speed with which it is broken down to glucose and thus hits the blood stream. Glucose has a value of 100 and water of 0. Any food with a GI below around 50 will thus be a good choice if you want high levels of concentration, focus and alertness.

Any food with a GI rating below around 50 is a good choice.

GI ratings of common food

Choose these...		Instead of these	
Apples	38	Chocolate bar	68
Basmati rice	58	White rice	87
Carrot	39	Potato (mashed)	73
Spaghetti	40	Jacket potato	85
All Bran	44	Cornflakes	83
Pita	57	Croissant	67
Yoghurt	36	Ice cream	61

Carbs – your daily fuel

Because carbohydrates can make you sleepy as they promote release of the neurotransmitter serotonin, it's wise to eat large amounts of carbs in the evening. During the day, concentrate on eating smaller quantities (about a fist size) of slow-releasing wholegrains (pasta, bread, rice) at each meal – wholegrain products are more slowly broken down.

However, you can safely eat lots and lots of vegetables (at least three portions and preferably around six) throughout the day. Vegetables are unrefined carbohydrate foods.

Eat fat and protein with your carbohydrates as this, too, slows down their breakdown and release into the bloodstream. For instance, a little oil or butter with bread, or cheese grated on pasta rather than on its own. There will be more of what to eat, when, to maximise your brain power in the following chapters.

Chapter 2
Brain-boosting Nutrients

When it comes to mental performance, you are what you eat, it seems.

We all know that when our stomach is rumbling with hunger we just don't have the ability to concentrate fully on the task in hand. And, at the other extreme, most of us have experienced that mental (and physical) slump after a big meal, when all we want to do is lie down and have a good snooze. Not the best state in which to whiz through the cryptic crossword, or brainstorm that work problem, or sit a physics exam.

But the brain is influenced by far more than how empty (or full) our stomach is. What we fill it with is crucial. It relies upon a perfect symphony of nutrients to make really sweet (and clever) music. We can see this in research on newborns. Studies show that bigger-birthweight babies may end up with higher IQs than lighter babies. It's thought the difference comes down to good nutrition in the womb.

Experts continue to debate the nature – or basis – of IQ. It's thought to be attributable largely to genes, and be influenced by social interaction, upbringing, our parents' involvement with us as children – did they play with us, read to us and so on. Birth order is also thought to play a role – first children tend on average to have a slightly higher IQ than subsequent children.

But what's making nutritionists really excited these days is that increasing numbers of studies concur that diet plays a crucial role in concentration, mental agility and learning ability.

For example, one report published in 2005 in the Journal of Nutrition and Food Science reviewed extensive research on the effect of nutrition on mental functions of children and adolescents. It concluded that 'nutrition has potent effects on brain function.' And that '… protein, iron, iodine and the consumption of breakfast all impact on a child's learning capability and behaviour. Moreover, recent research has identified additional, potent roles of micronutrients, such as essential fatty acids, minerals and vitamins in the prevention of learning and behavioural disorders.'

Your mind, then, like your body, is a finely tuned machine that requires sufficient amounts of the best kind of fuel in order to work optimally. That means filling it with the right balance of protein, carbohydrates and fats, and ensuring the diet includes good amounts of essential vitamins and minerals.

We have seen how the right kind of slower-releasing (complex) carbohydrates such as wholegrains and lean protein help provide the body and brain with a good supply of energy (see chapter 1 page 15).

Here we'll be looking at how vitamins and minerals are involved in brain function, and how ensuring a regular supply of vital nutrients is fundamental if we're to reach our full mental capacity.

Vitamins

There's not much you can do to alter your genes, but there's a lot you can do to make the most of the brains you were born with. Namely, nourish them.

That means ensuring you're getting a good balance of the vitamins and minerals you need to keep all your cells working as efficiently as possible.

Take vitamins, for example. Without all the 13 key vitamins, your body – and brain – can't function optimally. That's why a balanced diet it so important.

Vitamins are important because they're involved in processes such as growth, development, the release of energy from foods, the use of energy by your muscles, and to help protect your cells from free radical damage, caused by everyday nasties from pollution to sunlight, and even stress.

Vitamins are also needed to make the enzymes (or proteins) that regulate all the chemical reactions in our body, from digesting food to manufacturing those all-important neurotransmitters.

There are two main groups of vitamins – water-soluble vitamins (such as vitamin C and B vitamins) and fat-soluble vitamins. 'Water-soluble' means they dissolve in water, so don't remain in the body for long (excesses are lost in bodily fluids such as urine etc), so you need regular amounts of them. These vitamins are more vulnerable to cooking, processing, storage and general food preparation.

The other vitamins (A, D, E and K) are fat-soluble. That means they dissolve in fat, so are able to remain in your body's stores for longer.

There are recommended daily amounts of these vitamins, known as RNIs (Reference Nutrient Intake). If you're following a well balanced diet, the wide variety of foods you consume should provide all the vitamins you need to meet these requirements.

Vitamins for a healthy brain

Vitamin A

Vitamin A (otherwise known as retinol) is a fat-soluble vitamin which is stored mainly in your liver.

It's found in animal sources such as meat, fish and eggs – especially liver. Betacarotene (found in orange and leafy green vegetables such as carrots and squash, spinach and broccoli) is converted to vitamin A in the body.

It's important for the brain because it's involved in making some of the protein 'blocks' which are used in building and repairing our body's cells. This vitamin is also important for efficient eyesight (it helps us to see in the dark), the immune system, the growth and development of tissues and of bones, and for a balanced reproductive system.

Very high intakes during pregnancy may be linked to birth defects, so pregnant women are advised to avoid taking supplements and eating liver.

Betacarotene has a powerful antioxidant action in the body, helping to protect the cell membranes, proteins and DNA from damage.

According to the 2003 National Diet and Nutrition Survey, 10% of women aged 25–34 and 15% of those aged 19–24 are thought to have below recommended intakes.

Where can I get it?

Good sources of vitamin A (retinol) include milk, cheese, butter, herring and margarine. Carotenes are found in orange fruits and veg including mangoes and apricots, and dark leafy veg, and milk.

Vitamin B1

Also known as thiamin, vitamin B1 is a water-soluble vitamin which is vital for brain function, and specifically for the transmission of certain nerve signals between the brain and spinal cord. It also helps the release of energy from carbohydrates and is vital for the function of the heart and for the nervous system.

Although deficiencies are rare in the Western world (beri beri is no longer found in the UK), a lack of thiamin affects the nervous system and has been linked to loss of appetite, anxiety, tiredness and poor sleep. Because your body doesn't store this vitamin for very long, it's important to get regular intakes.

High intakes of alcohol can interfere with the absorption of thiamin, which can affect brain function.

Where can I get it?

Best sources include wholegrains, nuts and meat (especially pork), bran, wholemeal bread, eggs.

Niacin

Otherwise known as vitamin B3, this vitamin is found in most foods, and is used by the body to release energy from foods, for normal functioning of the nervous and digestive systems, and for healthy skin. Your body can also make niacin from the amino acid tryptophan.

The more active you are, the higher your need for vitamin B3.

Although deficiencies of this vitamin (known as pellagra) are rare in the Western world, low levels can have an effect on your mental wellbeing and are linked to headaches, irritability, poor sleep, emotional anxiety and depression.

Where can I get it?

Good sources include meat and milk, fish, pulses, nuts.

Good sources of Vitamin A include milk, eggs and fish. Betacarotene, found in orange and green leafy vegetables, is converted to Vitamin A by the body.

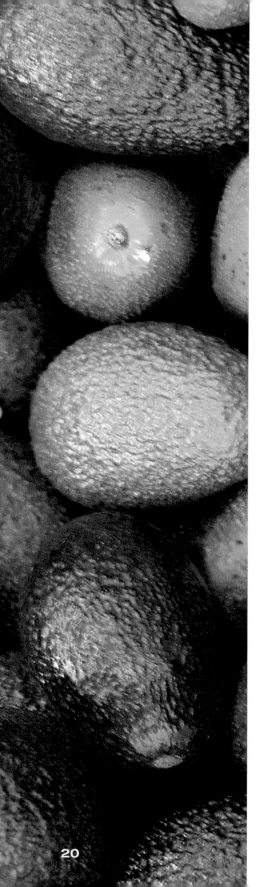

Pantothenic acid

Also known as vitamin B5, pantothenic acid is vital for the release of energy from food to nourish every cell in the body. It helps produce antibodies to help fight infection.

It's also involved in producing anti-stress hormones in the adrenal glands, and it plays a role in calming and soothing mind and body.

Pantothenic acid supplements have been found to help reduce fatigue and improve low moods and insomnia in people with poor diets.

Where can I get it?

Good sources include dried apricots and other dried fruits, nuts, sesame seeds, apples, avocados and calves' liver.

Vitamin B6

Vitamin B6 (also known as pyridoxine) is needed for the production of the feel-good neurotransmitter serotonin. (Those suffering from depression are often found to have low levels of this vitamin.) Supplements may also help those suffering from fatigue and tiredness.

It's thought vitamin B6 can also help balance hormones, which is why women suffering pre-menstrual symptoms such as depression and mood swings claim that vitamin B6 may help.

Your body also needs vitamin B6 to help release energy from protein, and to produce haemoglobin for red blood cells.

Where can I get it?

Fish, poultry, beef, eggs, wholegrains and nuts, and some fruits and vegetables.

Vitamin B12

This vitamin is vitally important for good brain health. It plays an essential role in keeping nerves healthy and is needed to create the myelin sheath which surrounds nerve cells, and for the transmission of nerve impulses – such as the feel-good substances serotonin and dopamine which help control our sleep patterns and moods.

Vitamin B12 is also important for the formation and maintenance of blood, and is vital for normal growth.

Vitamin B12 supplements are often used to help fight fatigue.

As it's found predominantly in animal produce, vegans are recommended to include B12 fortified foods (such as breakfast cereals and yeast extract) or take a B complex/multivitamin supplement to avoid deficiency, which could lead to anaemia and neurological damage.

Where can I get it?

Vitamin B12 is found in meat and fish, dairy products, eggs, yeast extract and fortified breakfast cereals.

Folic acid (folate)

Folic acid is involved in the metabolism of protein, and to help balance levels of the amino acid homocysteine, high levels of which increase your risk of stroke and heart disease.

It's also needed for cell division and for the formation of DNA.

Folic acid is involved in the development of the nervous system, and it is particularly important for neural tube development in the foetus in the first three months of pregnancy. (That's why pregnant women or women who are planning a pregnancy are advised to take a daily 400mcg supplement.)

A lack of folate in the diet may lead to anaemia and tiredness. It's best absorbed when taken with foods rich in B vitamins.

Folic acid supplements have also been found to improve memory and to speed up the brain's information processing abilities. Raised homocysteine levels are also linked with low moods and depression, so folate may play an important role in helping regulate mood.

Where can I get it?

Best sources include dark green leafy veg such as spinach and Brussels sprouts, fortified breakfast cereals, asparagus, peas, broccoli and some nuts.

You can get 200mcg from one portion of lentils – or from a 40g serving of fortified breakfast cereal (100mcg) and from one 80g serving of cooked spinach (97mcg) – or from one slice of honeydew melon (50mcg), one glass of orange juice (40mcg) and two slices of wholemeal toast with yeast extract (120mcg).

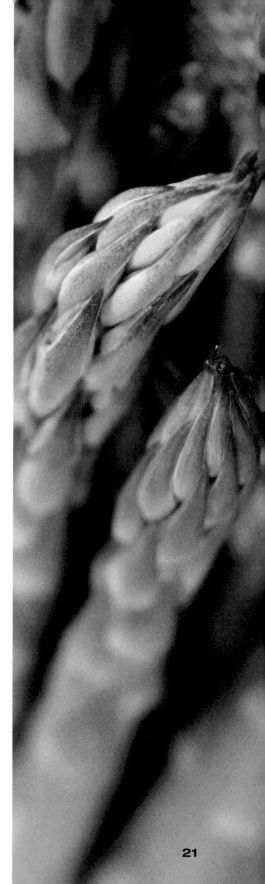

Vitamin C

Vitamin C (otherwise known as ascorbic acid) is a water-soluble antioxidant vitamin needed to produce collagen (the protein in connective tissue). This is vital for all cells which make up skin, teeth, bones and gums, as well as the tiny capillaries which transport blood in the body and brain. It aids healing and is vital for the immune system, and helps mop up damage wrought by free radicals.

Vitamin C is also needed to help facilitate the absorption of iron from foods (particularly plant sources).

It's easily destroyed by cooking, and stress hormones in the body may deplete vitamin C levels. We need good amounts every day as it can't be stored in the body.

Where can I get it?

Best sources are berries, citrus fruit, tomatoes, peppers and broccoli.

Vitamin E

Vitamin E is a fat-soluble vitamin and an antioxidant which helps neutralise free radicals and protect the lipids (or fats) in cell walls against damage. It's involved in maintaining healthy skin, nerves, muscles and blood cells. It's thought to have anti-inflammatory effects and to help boost the immune system. Vitamin E has been linked to the reduction of certain cancers and heart disease.

Although it's fat-soluble, vitamin E doesn't stay in the body for long, which means we need regular supplies.

Some studies have shown that vitamin E may help slow down the progression of the neurological condition Parkinson's disease.

Where can I get it?

Best sources include nuts, avocados, vegetable oils e.g. sunflower, green leafy veg, and seeds such as sunflower seeds.

Other vitamins for good health

Vitamin B2

Vitamin B2 is also known as riboflavin, and, like thiamin, it's very important for the release of energy from food, especially from fats and protein. It's also needed for the transport and metabolism of iron, for healthy skin, and for the production of normal mucous membranes. Low intakes may cause cracked skin around the mouth and nose, and national survey data suggests that 'significant numbers of teenagers and young women have low intakes of riboflavin'.

Where can I get it?

Milk and dairy products, fortified breakfast cereals, eggs and yeast extracts, fish such as mackerel.

Biotin

This B vitamin plays a role alongside the other B vitamins in helping the body convert proteins, carbs and fats into energy for the body.

Where can I get it?

It's found in most foods, including eggs, liver and yeast extract, and nuts.

Vitamin D

Vitamin D is manufactured by the action of sunlight on the skin, and is used for helping control the absorption of calcium in the body, which is vital for bones and teeth. Lack of vitamin D can cause rickets and bone problems, and certain groups in the UK (such as Asian women and Asian children) are thought to be more at risk of deficiency.

Where can I get it?

Food sources include oily fish, eggs, butter and meat. Margarine is fortified with vitamin D (by law).

Vitamin K

Vitamin K is involved in the clotting of blood and in the production of proteins. Deficiency is rare in adults but is sometimes seen in newborn babies, which is why supplements are often given to babies at birth.

Where can I get it?

It's made in the body by bacteria in the intestines, and it's also available in dark green leafy veg such as cabbage, and Brussels sprouts.

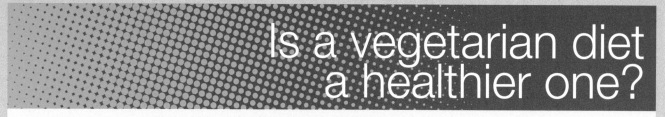

Is a vegetarian diet a healthier one?

It certainly can be. Vegetarians have 30% less heart disease, up to 40% less cancer, tend to be slimmer and have lower blood pressure than meat eaters.

It's true that some nutrition experts warn that it may be harder for veggies to get all their vital vitamins and minerals – particularly iron – but the British Nutrition Foundation's studies show no notable difference between vegetarians and meat eaters in terms of iron deficiency.

The key is to make sure you eat a variety of foods. The Vegetarian Society Balance of Good Health recommends five portions of fruit & veg a day; five portions of starchy food such as potatoes, wholegrain bread or cereals; two to three portions of calcium-rich dairy or soya foods; two to three portions of protein-rich foods such as pulses, nuts, seeds, eggs, tofu, vegetable or mycoprotein; and small amounts of 'good' fat – up to about three portions a day.

Good fats include olive oil or sunflower oil, preferably non-hydrogenated. A serving is about one level teaspoon of oil or spread. Nuts and seeds also contain 'good fats'. Aim to get no more than 30% of your daily calorie intake from fats – that's about 70g a day – avoiding high-fat dairy products and processed foods containing dairy fats and hydrogenated vegetable fats, and using olive or nut oils for cooking purposes.

In terms of the vitamins and minerals that may be harder for a vegetarian to come by, vitamin B12 can be obtained from eggs, milk, fortified soya products, and yeast extract. And calcium is available in good amounts in sesame seeds or tahini (an ingredient of hummus).

Lentils and wholegrains provide zinc, and leafy green veg contains vitamins A, B group, C and K.

The best sources of iron are beans, eggs, tofu, spinach, cabbage, wholegrains, dried fruit and parsley. To improve iron absorption, eat with a food rich in vitamin C.

Getting more from your vitamins

Not all vitamins come in a form which is easily accessible by the body. And certain vitamins are more easily absorbed if they have other key nutrients at their disposal. In order to get more from your vitamins, aim to try some clever teamwork in your daily diet.

For example, ideally aim to drink orange juice with your iron-rich cereal, or green, leafy veg or steak. Vitamin C aids the absorption of iron.

One study from the American Journal of Clinical Nutrition (2004) found that you'll absorb more of the disease-fighting antioxidants lycopene, betacarotene and alpha carotene from salads if you eat them with a bit of fat. So try adding a dash of olive oil to your salad rather than fat-free dressing or than crunching them raw.

Fruit salad for pud? You'll absorb more vitamin E from your fruits if you sprinkle some seeds or nuts over them, as fats can help you absorb fat-soluble nutrients.

Another study by the Institute of Food Research found that mushrooms and broccoli are tougher cancer beaters when they're eaten together as their powerful nutrients sulphorane and selenium work best together. Try mixing them in a tasty stir fry.

- **Other good partners include red meat and sweet potatoes or carrots.** These veggies are rich in betacarotene which can help absorption of the iron. Try a shepherd's pie with sweet potatoes instead of regular ones.
- **Eat plenty of leafy green veg, peas and asparagus.** Incorporating good amounts of folate (folic acid) in your diet helps to protect your body's stores of iron.
- **Cut back on coffee.** Large quantities of caffeine can affect the absorption of B vitamins in the body. Stick to one cup or try switching to decaff.
- **Don't drink tea with meals.** Tea can reduce the absorption of iron in the body. So stick to food-free tea breaks.
- **Team shredded wheat with milk alongside your orange juice.** Vitamin C works best in conjunction with calcium (found in milk) and magnesium (in cereals).

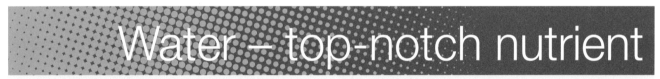

Water – top-notch nutrient

Your blood is over 80% water, and your blood supply is a supersonic transport system; it brings nutrients to your brain and helps rid the body of toxins.

That's why adequate hydration is crucial to a hard-working brain. Being dehydrated can all too easily drain your mental resources.

According to a study at Leeds University, schoolchildren with the best results were those who drank up to eight glasses of water a day. (For more tips on good hydration see page 43.)

Minerals

Minerals are nutrients (inorganic substances) that the body needs in tiny amounts to help perform vital functions. They're required for making and maintaining bones and for healthy levels of body fluids. But they're also vital for the brain in helping the nerves to make neurotransmitters, the chemical messengers which transmit impulses between nerves and the brain.

We require certain minerals in larger amounts – such as calcium, magnesium, phosphorus, sodium, potassium and chloride. Other 'trace' minerals are needed in smaller quantities, but they're still just as vital for good health. They are iron, zinc, iodine, fluoride, selenium and copper.

Although most people are not deficient in many of these minerals, data from the National Diet and Nutrition Surveys show that teenagers, young adults and older people are low in certain minerals such as potassium, magnesium and zinc.

It's thought that numbers of women of childbearing age and teenage girls may also be deficient in minerals such as iron and calcium.

Calcium

Calcium is important for building bones and teeth. A small fraction (1%) of calcium is also found in your body's tissues. Here it plays a role in regulating fluids. It's also vital for intracellular signalling for nerve and muscle function. Calcium is thought to work alongside magnesium at regulating sleep and mood.

Calcium works in tandem with vitamin D (produced by the body when exposed to sunlight, and found in oily fish and butter).

Where can I get it?

Best sources include dairy products such as cheese, wholemilk, yoghurt. It's also found in bony fish (such as sardines), and tofu and figs.

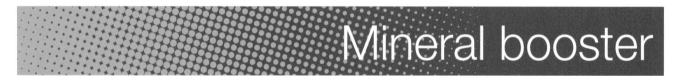

Mineral booster

How to get more calcium in your diet? Try adding fat-free powdered milk to your mashed potatoes, casseroles, soups and sauces. One 220ml (8 fl oz) pot of yoghurt has 100mg more calcium than the same amount of milk. Non-dairy calcium sources include green leafy vegetables, baked beans, bony fish and dried fruit.

Magnesium

Magnesium is important for energy metabolism, for muscle function and for healthy bones and teeth. It also aids the transmission of nerves. It's also involved in the transportation of insulin, so plays a role in the balancing of blood sugar levels. A lack of magnesium is linked with nerve disorders, palpitations and weak muscles, fatigue and restlessness.

Where can I get it?

Magnesium is found in leafy green vegetables, wholegrains and nuts, seeds and bananas.

Potassium

This mineral works in tandem with sodium to regulate your body's fluid levels within the cells and to maintain healthy blood pressure. It is needed for the transmission of messages between nerves and muscles.

Where can I get it?

Fruits and veg are a rich source – for example bananas, oranges, watercress and spinach, avocados – and nuts and seeds. It's also found in dried fruit and milk.

Sodium

Found in your bones and also in your body's fluids, sodium is vital for maintaining the balance of water in the body. It helps maintain healthy muscles, and to aid absorption of nutrients in the intestines. Too much salt is linked to high blood pressure and stroke (see page 73 for tips on keeping your salt intake under control).

Phosphorus

You need phosphorus to help release the energy in your cells, for healthy bones and teeth, and for the structure of cell membranes (in phospholipids found in every cell in the body). It's also important for the absorption of nutrients.

Where can I get it?

It's available in milk and dairy products, seafood, poultry and meat.

Iron

Your body needs iron for the formation of haemoglobin in blood cells, which transports oxygen around the body and to your brain. Iron is also needed for energy production, and for a healthy immune system.

Figures show that as many as two out of five women have inadequate levels of iron. Low levels cause fatigue, tiredness and can lead to anaemia.

There's good evidence to show that getting enough iron in your diet can boost concentration. One study from the University of the State of Mexico found that children deficient in iron had lower IQ levels than children with sufficient intakes of iron, who also performed better on comprehension tests.

Where can I get it?

Eggs, lean meat, green leafy veg, baked beans, fortified breakfast cereals.

Boron is a mineral important for healthy bones and teeth. It's also been found to be valuable for maintaining mental alertness; one US study found that people with low levels of boron in their diet had poorer attention levels, dexterity and short-term memory, and were less adept at performing certain mental tasks in tests. Best sources of boron are vegetables, fruit and nuts.

Trace elements

Manganese

Manganese is a trace element which your body needs for energy metabolism and for healthy bones. It's involved in maintaining healthy nerves and helps balance blood sugar levels. Manganese is needed for the formation of an anti-oxidant enzyme which helps protects the cells.

Where can I get it?

It's found in wholegrains and nuts, and, in smaller quantities, in fruits and veg, and in tea.

Zinc

Zinc is vital for a healthy immune system, and for healing wounds. It's involved in maintaining cell membranes, and in protecting your cells from damage.

Your body also needs it for sexual development and reproduction (it helps men produce healthy sperm). Plus it helps keep your senses such as taste and smell working efficiently, and can boost the growth of your nails and hair.

A deficiency is linked to neurological impairment, and fatigue and anxiety.

Where can I get it?

Best sources are red meat, liver, eggs, dairy products, seafoods, pumpkin seeds.

Tip: zinc is absorbed better by the body if you eat protein sources as part of the same meal.

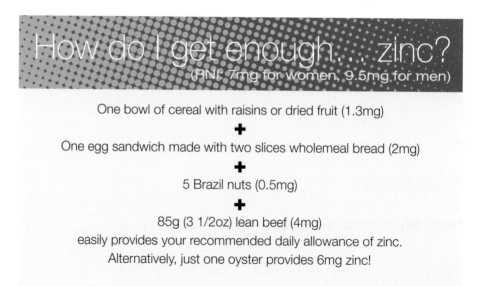

How do I get enough... zinc?
(RNI: 7mg for women, 9.5mg for men)

One bowl of cereal with raisins or dried fruit (1.3mg)
+
One egg sandwich made with two slices wholemeal bread (2mg)
+
5 Brazil nuts (0.5mg)
+
85g (3 1/2oz) lean beef (4mg)
easily provides your recommended daily allowance of zinc.
Alternatively, just one oyster provides 6mg zinc!

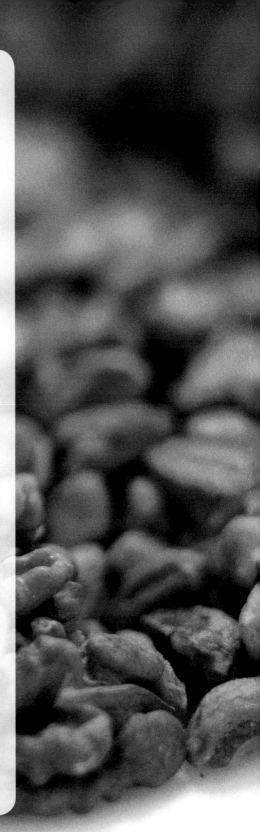

Iodine

Iodine is used to make thyroid hormones which help regulate our metabolic rate, and for normal neurological development. Deficiency is uncommon, but it's thought that about 1 in 8 young women have lower than recommended intakes.

Where can I get it?

It's found in saltwater fish and shellfish, and in dairy products.

Selenium

Selenium plays an important role in helping to neutralise free radicals in the body, and so protect our cells. We also need it for normal growth and development and for the production of hormones. It's involved in the production of sperm and for prostate health.

Where can I get it?

Good sources include Brazil nuts, dairy products, avocados, sunflower seeds, wholemeal bread.

Copper

Copper is involved in nerve function and the release of energy, and helps the body absorb iron from food.

Where can I get it?

It's found in calves' liver, seafood such as oysters, sunflower seeds and nuts, and cocoa.

Chromium

It's thought to be involved in the regulation of blood sugar levels. Some anecdotal evidence suggests chromium may play a role in helping reduce sweet cravings.

Where can I get it?

Red meat, wholegrains, nuts, beans such as mung beans.

Molybdenum

It plays a role in helping the body use the energy from food, and iron. It also helps keep nerves healthy and is important for mental alertness.

Where can I get it?

Liver, lentils, wholemeal bread, kidney beans.

Fats

Fat is a word that weight-aware and health-conscious people have learned to fear. But the truth is fats are absolutely vital to good nutrition and crucial to brain function. It's thought that the brain is about 60% fat (after water is removed) – attributable to the myelin sheath that surrounds the brain cells, which is itself about 75% fat. The trick is to familiarise yourself with the right – and wrong – fats to put into your body.

So what do fats do that makes them so important for a healthy brain?

For a start they play a role in memory, and they help make vital hormones and also influence mood.

They also help keep the immune system working, and are important for healthy blood circulation.

The body needs fat in the diet in order to absorb fat-soluble vitamins A, D, E and K, to build cell membranes and provide 'essential' fats that the body cannot make. Healthy fat stores also help insulate the body, and cushion bones and joints.

But it's important to get a good balance of the right fats. And to make sure we never cut fats from our diet completely – even if we're hoping to shed a few pounds. Instead we should aim for most of our fat to be the mono-unsaturated or polyunsaturated kind, while avoiding saturated fats as far as possible.

Here's your guide to good and bad fats.

Good fats

Polyunsaturated fats

There are two families of polyunsaturated fats, each headed by a 'parent' essential fatty acid; linoleic acid (the omega-6 family), and alpha-linoleic acid (omega-3 family).

These fatty acids are needed for growth, cell membranes, and to produce eicosanoids – chemical messengers that help regulate blood clotting, blood pressure and immunity.

Omega 3s: Brain food

We're constantly being told how good these fats are for our body and our brain. Omega-3 fatty acids are found in oily fish such as sardines, mackerel, fresh tuna and salmon, trout and herring, pumpkin seeds, flaxseeds and flax-seed oil, soya oil and omega-3-enriched eggs.

There are two types of omega-3 fatty acids – EPA (eicosapentaenoic acid) and DHA (docosahexaenoic acid). Experts say they're easily absorbed into cell membranes, which means they have far-reaching benefits; they've been found to help keep the brain healthy and have a positive effect on mood, as well as being beneficial for the heart, joints and even the skin.

Benefits for the brain

- Fish oils help strengthen your brain cell membranes and improve brain function by boosting blood flow.
- They are particularly beneficial to a foetus's developing brain; pregnant women are encouraged to up their intake of oily fish in the last few months of pregnancy. Breastfeeding mothers, too, are advised to get plenty of fish oils in their diet to maximise their baby's brain development.
- Children given healthy amounts of omega-3 fatty acids have been found to do better at school. And ongoing research indicates that symptoms of dyslexia and hyperactivity in children have been helped with supplements of EPA and DHA.
- It's thought the DHA in fish oils may help stave off dementia, help memory and alertness, and improve concentration.
- Fish oils can also be an effective mood booster. Research published in the American Journal of Psychiatry found that fish-oil supplements helped six out of ten people suffering from depression.

Omega 3's other benefits

Many studies show that omega-3 fatty acids are important for heart health; they've been linked to lowered blood pressure, and a reduced risk of stroke and heart attack. One study from the University of Missouri-Columbia found that fish oils helped lower triglyceride levels by 38%. (Triglycerides are linked to high blood pressure, and, like cholesterol, are bad for your heart.) An Italian study of cardiac patients found that people who took 1g of fish oil each day were 45% less likely to die of sudden, heart-related causes. Fish-oil supplements are often recommended for people with high cholesterol or family history of heart disease.

Omega-3 fatty acids found in fish oils are naturally anti-inflammatory and can help with rheumatoid arthritis. Research published in the medical journal Drug Discovery Today showed that taking fish-oil supplements can slow down the destruction of cartilage and alleviate joint inflammation.

Skin foods

If you're after an inexpensive beauty treatment, fish oils may be your answer. Nutrition experts say omega 3s can boost the elasticity and muscle tone of your skin, helping to keep it youthful for longer. And studies show psoriasis patients taking fish oil experienced reduced symptoms of flakiness and irritation.

Disease fighters
Research from the University of Southern California found that omega 3s may help reduce your risk of breast cancer, and other studies show that eating fish may help reduce colon cancer.

How much do we need?

Best food sources of oily fish are salmon, mackerel, herring or sardines; nutritionists say we should aim to eat about two portions of fish a week, one of which should be oily fish. Pregnant or breastfeeding women should avoid shark, swordfish and marlin, which may have high mercury levels.

Alternatively, get the goodness of omega-3 fatty acids in supplement form; fish oils are available in capsules, tablets or as liquid. If you're not a fan of fish, or are vegetarian, eat plant foods such as flaxseeds or flaxseed oil, walnuts, or organic milk and cheese. Seeds, soybeans and tofu are also good sources.

Omega 6s

These fatty acids include linoleic acid and gamma linoleic acid (GLA) which are found in sunflower oil, soya, corn and safflower oils. It's also found in evening primrose oil and borage (starflower) oil.

Getting the right balance

Omega-6 fatty acids are easier to find in foods than omega 3s, and most of us eat too much omega 6 in relation to omega 3s. This results in an imbalance of prostaglandins, 'mini hormones' which are responsible for controlling blood clotting, inflammation and the immune system.

We should be aiming for a ration of no more than five times the amount of omega 6s to omega 3s (most diets are a ratio of 10:1).

Good combinations of the two can be found naturally in sunflower seeds, sesame, pumpkin seeds, hemp seed and linseed (flax).

Mono-unsaturated fats

These fats are good at raising levels of good cholesterol, and lowering bad levels, and can also reduce the risk of heart disease. It's thought they may help cut your cancer risk too.

Olive oil is the best known, but these fats are available in rapeseed oil too, and in avocados, sunflower and sesame seeds, soya oil and nuts such as peanuts, almonds and cashews.

Extra virgin

According to US anti-ageing guru Dr Michael Roizen (www.realage.com) extra virgin olive oil has a higher concentration of cancer-fighting antioxidants – omega-3 fatty acids and squalene (a compound which may help prevent colon cancer).

Extra virgin means the acidity is less than 1% – the oil came from the first pressing of olives and the olives were cold-pressed, a process that preserves the nutrients and keeps the oil flavourful. The darker the colour, the deeper the flavour.

Bad fats

Saturated fats

These include butter, lard, block margarine and cooking fat (they're the fats that are solid at room temperature). They're mainly found in animal products such as meat and dairy foods, and in pastries, cakes, biscuits and deep fried foods.

Experts tell us that too many saturates have been found to raise levels of harmful cholesterol in the blood, which can be deposited in the arteries, leading to heart disease.

These fats raise levels of bad low-density lipoprotein (LDL) blood cholesterol and cause a fatty cholesterol-rich build-up on blood vessels which restricts blood flow to your cells.

By cutting down on butter, fatty meat, eggs, full fat dairy products, junk food and processed foods such as cakes, pastries, biscuits and pies, you'll reduce your intake of bad fats.

Cutting your intake of saturated fat can reduce women's risk of breast cancer, according to a recent study reported in the *Lancet*. Their research showed that women who eat more than 90g of fat per day are twice as likely to develop breast cancer as those who eat very low levels of fat – 40g or less fat each day.

UK health experts suggest women eat no more than 70g of fat each day but by keeping your intake of saturated fats to a minimum (10–20g a day), and making sure you stick to the healthiest kinds – found in nuts, olive and vegetable oils and avocados, and oily fish – you can reduce your risk.

The really bad guys – Trans fatty acids

These actually start off as unsaturated fats but become what we know as 'trans fatty acids' when hydrogen gas is added to vegetable oils to make them more solid. This also increases their shelf life, and they're found in processed foods such as cakes, biscuits and other convenience foods.

They're considered more harmful than saturated fats, and studies have shown that trans fats raise levels of bad LDL cholesterol in your body to a greater extent than saturated fats while also reducing the levels of good HDL cholesterol, something saturated fat doesn't do.

Researchers at the University of Oxford recently called for food labels to list trans fats as well as cholesterol and saturated fat to help reduce coronary heart disease.

A recent analysis found a 2% increase in the energy intake from trans fatty acids was associated with a 23% increase in the occurrence of coronary heart disease. In fact, the authors noted that the harmful effects of trans fatty acids were seen even when intake was really low, only 3% of total daily energy intake (20–60 calories), about 2–7 g for a person consuming 2,000 calories per day.

The UK Food Standards Agency (FSA) believe that mandatory addition of the content of saturated fat and trans fatty acids to nutrition labels would help people to make healthier food choices that could lower LDL concentrations and reduce the risk of coronary heart disease.

The FSA is currently campaigning for a revision of the European directive that governs the content and format of nutrition labels on foods marketed in the United Kingdom and other European countries, so that these fats are labelled.

Eat your fats

Your body needs one to two daily servings of essential fatty acids and mono-unsaturated fats each day for energy, eye function, brain-power and healthy skin and hair. Fats are also needed to absorb fat-soluble vitamins A, D, E and K which are important for vision and strong bones, and to help fight disease.

Here's where to get it:
80g (one-quarter to one-half) of an avocado
One tablespoon of olive or rapeseed oil
10g (half an ounce) butter
2 tablespoons of low-fat mayo
2 tablespoons sunflower or pumpkin seeds
4–6 walnuts
3–4 tablespoons hummus
150g oily fish such as sardines or mackerel

How much fat do I need?

Aim to keep your fat intake to no more than 25% of your daily calories – about 50g of fat a day, and no more than 70g. Of this, no more than 20g should be saturated fat.

Fibre

Fibre is a vital part of your brain-boosting healthy diet because adequate amounts of it help keep your digestive system in good working order. Constipation can deplete your energy levels and leave you feeling lacklustre.

The good news is you don't have to eat buckets of bran to get your daily quota. As well as being good for your gut and reducing cancer risk, fibre's also great for regulating your metabolism; it's digested more slowly than other nutrients so it can prevent insulin spikes you often get from sugary foods which encourage your body to lay down fat.

Aim for a cereal with at least 7g fibre per serving, say experts – eating cereal is the best way to get fibre in a smaller package.

Although high intakes of wheat bran can deplete your levels of minerals, you can get plenty of fibre from wholegrains, fruits and veg. Soluble fibre is found in oatmeal, beans and certain fruits – such as kiwi fruits, raspberries, kumquats and blackcurrants – and is especially protective against heart disease. It slows glucose absorption in your bloodstream and helps lower cholesterol levels.

You can get your recommended intake of fibre (that's about 18g) from one bowl of bran flakes plus one apple plus beans on wholewheat toast (100g beans).

Vitamin C savers

- Cook fruit and veggies in the least possible amount of water; when you cook 100g veg in 400ml of water, you lose 90% of the vitamin C. Reverse this – one part water to four parts veggies, you retain 50% of the vitamin C.
- Roast or boil root veggies (carrots, potatoes and sweet potatoes) in their skins and you save almost 100% of their vitamin C.

Protein and brain chemicals

Neurotransmitters are made from the amino acids found in proteins such as meat, poultry, fish and cheese.

Here are the three key transmitters and where to get them

1. Acetylcholine: responsible for your memory, and involved with voluntary movement and muscles. Good sources include eggs, milk, cheese, fish, meat and vegetables (especially cruciferous veg such as broccoli, cabbage and cauliflower).
2. Dopamine: important for movement, learning, emotional arousal. Good sources include proteins such as meat, milk, nuts, soya products.
3. Serotonin: involved in sleep, mood, appetite and sensitivity. Also is involved in pleasurable feelings. Good sources include carbohydrate-rich foods such as pasta, starchy veg, potatoes.

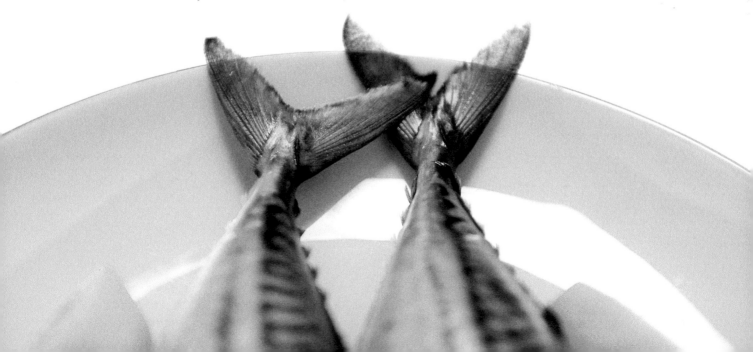

You and your memory
Why do we start to forget?

How sharp is your memory these days? Are you able to retain facts and figures, telephone numbers and your bank PIN numbers? Do you ever have days when you just can't recall names and important information?

It is common to lose memory as we get older, but that does not mean it is inevitable.

We can do a great deal to make sure that our memory remains razor sharp until the day we die. It's never too late to start sharpening your memory but the best time to start is yesterday!

That's because we now know that the brain begins to age at a much earlier age than originally thought. Indeed, some researchers believe that our memory begins to decline not long after the age that our brain stops growing – around the early to mid-twenties! Certainly, by our mid-thirties, memory loss may have started for some of us, even if its only manifestation is the occasional 'what on earth is his name again?'.

Why are some people more susceptible? The reasons are sometimes genetic, but mostly due to lifestyle.

That's encouraging. It means we can do much to prevent memory loss. University of Kentucky research shows that only about 5% of memory impairment is due to brain disorders such as Alzheimer's. Stress, depression, lack of exercise and poor nutrition are far more common causes.

Memory loss is due to several factors

- **Diminished blood circulation.** Your brain has a high demand for nutrients and oxygen, and it receives them via the blood carried to it by a vast circulation system. Just as with any other arteries in the body, these blood vessels can become 'furred up' if you smoke or eat a diet that is not beneficial to the circulatory system (for example, too high in 'bad' fats or sugar). This is the reason that exercise – improving lung function – has been proven to help the brain and keep it young. It's also thought that exercise leads to the release of nerve growth factor that actually promotes the growth of new brain cells.
- **Genetic medical conditions.** There is a family component to Alzheimer's disease and some people begin to show signs of this illness as early as their thirties.
- **Trauma.** Accidents or repeated injury (through, for example, boxing) cause damages to the insulation of the nerve cells which in turn leads to memory loss and less efficient processing of information. Even seemingly unimportant accidents can lead to memory loss decades later, which is why it's important to wear helmets when engaging in sports at all ages, not just childhood.

But studies have shown that memory training can make a real difference to the ageing of the brain. Age does not affect the amount of material you can absorb in a given period, or your ability to learn a new skill.

MEMORY TRAINING
Build a better memory.

- **Focus on one thing at a time.** The more distractions around you when you're laying down a memory, the more chances you'll forget it. So when you're reading info you want to retain, it's best to switch off TV or the radio.

- **Listen and repeat.** We hear, but we don't always listen. Next time you want to remember something, such as a new colleague's name, really pay attention when you're introduced. Say their name as soon as you can out loud to cement it into your memory. Then pause, and repeat it again, even if it's to yourself. 'Repeat, pause, repeat' is simple, but it works. Similarly, if you're given info you want to be sure to remember, immediately you've got it, say 'let me just check I've got this right …' and repeat the information straight back.

- **Sensory stimulation helps.** We often remember moments of high negative emotional intensity vividly and that's because we automatically notice everything that is going on around us when we feel ourselves in danger. The more senses you can 'rope in' to help you cement a memory, the more likely you'll be able to recall it later. So don't just notice the beautiful sunset, take note of how the sand feels under your feet, the sound of waves on the beach, and champagne bubbles on your tongue. Anchoring our memories in the sensory world fires off more neurones in our brain and keeps the memory fresher.

- **Take a nap.** When learning new information or a skill, research shows that taking a nap after the initial learning experience improves your chance of retaining the memory better than if you had just carried on without sleeping.

Slowing the signs of ageing

Keep your brain flexible by stretching it.

WIDEN your horizons

The more you keep learning, the better your 'cognitive functioning'; in other words, the more efficient your brain. When we learn something new, neurones are fired in unfamiliar parts of the brain and this literally grows the brain. It's easier to learn Spanish when you're 6 than when you're 60, but that doesn't mean that a 60-year-old cannot do it. Every month, read or research on the internet a subject that interests you but that you know little about. Or set yourself a new study goal each year – a language, an instrument or a skill.

PUSH yourself

Another way to slow down the ageing process is to duplicate the process of learning to read. Teachers move on learner readers by asking them to read a page of a book. If the child can read it easily, the teacher discards it, but if she is getting one to three words wrong in every ten, that is likely to be the book the teacher will choose: it's pitched at the right level of difficulty, enough to stretch the child but not too difficult so she becomes discouraged.

This is almost exactly what research shows us adults should do to keep their brains active. You may love to whiz through your crossword, rejoicing in how quickly you complete it, but if you really want to test your brain, raise your game. Pick puzzles, crosswords or situations such as pub quizzes where you are right around 80% of the time and wrong about 20%. Research shows that this level keeps your brain sharp.

GO on holiday

Change your routine. Doing things differently keeps your brain flexible, better at thinking and better at retaining information. The most enjoyable way to do this is to travel to a different part of the world and immerse yourself in its culture, but you can get the same effects in other ways. Mix up your daily routine. Take a different route to work every day this week, see a movie you'd never think of seeing – perhaps in a foreign language – or shop in a totally different locale. Try to do something differently every day.

7 steps to a younger brain

- **Eat regularly.** Try three meals a day and two snacks, preferably. Lack of a steady flow of fuel has been shown to reduce memory in rat studies.
- **Eat oily fish once a week**, or take supplements of omega 3 or evening primrose oil.
- **Look to your lignans.** These nutrients, found in broccoli and berries, protect memory. Those eating 3oz of berries or 7oz of broccoli a day scored around 50% better in memory tests
- **Drink tea.** Green is good – four cups a day is linked to a reduced level of Alzheimer's – but black is fine, too, thanks to tea's high antioxidant levels.
- **Drink red wine rather than white wine.** It has been shown to keep your brain younger. But keep your intake moderate: too much alcohol weakens memory and cognition. Drinking one or two drinks a week gave a slight advantage over abstention in one study.
- **Start walking for 10 minutes a day**, working up to 45 minutes around three times a week. This has been shown to lead to a younger brain.
- **Be sociable.** Those who are involved in their community and keep in touch with friends and family are more likely to think young than those who become isolated as they grow older.
- **Consider supplementing with vitamins C and E.** Taken separately they make no difference but together they had the effect of preventing age-related decline in one large study.

Young brains: boosting babies' and toddlers' brain power

Experts say the toddler and pre-school years between three and five are a critical time for learning and development. The way we play and interact with young children, and what we feed them, has a significant impact on their brain.

Feed little brains

Good nutrition is vital to get the network of connections in the brain working at their full potential.

Recent Durham Sure Start trials have assessed the effects of fish-oil supplements on pre-school children. Researchers saw children whose learning skills went from being six months below their chronological age to absolutely normal in just three months. Some two-year-olds in the trial made leaps in their speech; many went from having a 25-word vocabulary to using whole sentences.

It's the omega-3 fatty acids in fish oils that are believed to help boost brain function by their positive action on the brain's neural transmitters. Researchers and parents noticed the children's concentration improving within a week of taking the supplements.

Experts recommend getting omega 3s from food rather than supplements. If you can get your child to eat oily fish (such as salmon, mackerel, herring or sardines) twice a week, then you're setting them up for life.

It's also important to ensure your child eats a healthy, balanced diet, and has sufficient amounts of iron in his diet. Iron deficiencies have been linked with delayed development or behaviour problems in young children. Good sources include red meat, leafy green veg, legumes such as beans, and wholegrain bread.

And try to steer your child away from additives. One government-funded study at the UK's Asthma and Allergy Research Centre found that certain food colours and preservatives cause hyperactive behaviour in as many as one in four young children. They recommend that all children would benefit from the removal of artificial food colourings from their diet.

Ones to avoid include tartrazine (E102), sunset yellow (E110), carmoisine (E122), ponceau 4R (E124) and the preservative sodium benzoate (E211). Start checking labels, and avoid fizzy drinks and sweets.

Boost little brains

Limit the television: researchers have found those who watch more than three hours a day are more likely to drop out of school without qualifications. And studies at the University of Washington in Seattle found that under-threes who watched the most television performed worst in reading and maths at tests at ages six and seven. Watching several hours of TV a day has also been linked with attention deficit disorder and poor concentration.

It's thought that the unnatural levels of stimulation and the flashing images can overstimulate young brains. US experts recommend that the under-twos do not watch any television at all. However, other experts argue that a limited amount of television or DVDs – as long as it is educational – can be beneficial to young minds.

It's thought that limited and supervised watching of TV and DVDs can be useful, because they may give children the opportunity to experience fantasy and stories. However the best advice is to sit and watch with your child so you can help offer explanations and be there to answer questions so it becomes an interactive and informative experience.

Chapter 3
Beat Your Cravings

Chocolate, anyone? Or how about a lovely cream cake?

We all know that the kind of food we eat has a knock-on effect on the way we feel. And we're also all too aware that the way we feel affects our choice of foods. Who hasn't reached for the biscuit tin or headed to the sweet shop for a large bar of chocolate during a bad day?

Many of us may become overwhelmed by our desire for a certain food – and go to great lengths to get it. Whereas desiring a certain food and indulging occasionally is perfectly healthy, trouble starts when the desire becomes out of control, or when we eat some of the desired food but we're not able to stop at one regular-sized portion.

We're discovering the impact that certain foods have on our brain. But there's more to consider. When we're preoccupied with food – wondering what to eat when, to save calories, or obsessively avoiding or bingeing on a certain food, or worrying about how to amend for a binge – our brain becomes fettered by anxieties, and just isn't free to focus on other matters, or roam productively. We're just not reaching our full mental potential when we're allowing our preoccupations with food to cloud our mind.

That said, most people do experience cravings at some time or other. Experts say that 98% of women have cravings compared with just 68% of men. One study in the International Journal of Eating Disorders assessed the cravings of 538 women and 506 men. They found that women's cravings were more likely to be linked to a negative mood – boredom, loneliness, depression – or occur when they were annoyed. Men's cravings were linked to a more positive mood. Other research has shown that women often tend to gravitate towards sweet snacks; men's cravings are more likely to be for savoury foods.

So why do we have cravings? There may be many different reasons, and several triggers. Do any of the following apply to you?

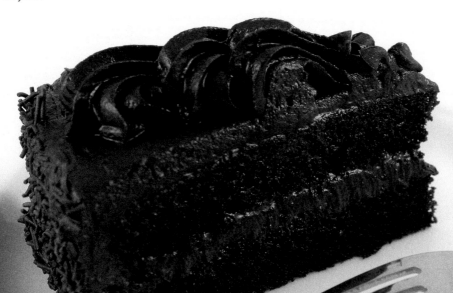

(Real) Hunger

Anyone who has ever slavishly tried to restrict their calorie intake – often bypassing breakfast and fasting until lunchtime – will be all too familiar with an overwhelming desire for food – or a certain type of food. These kinds of hunger pangs are completely natural.

When your body is low on fuel, the hunger signal starts in the hypothalamus – which then sends signals to other parts of the brain. These then emit chemical messengers which govern what we want to eat, and when we want to eat it.

However, when your blood sugar and your body's stores of carbohydrates (or glycogen) are low, the hypothalamus releases a chemical messenger neuropeptide Y (known as NPY). As this increases, your body's desires for sweet and starchy foods increase too. That's when you're lured to the biscuit tin or those chocolate bars.

The key is to keep your body satisfied by eating often – small meals every two to four hours can help keep hunger pangs at bay. Above all, don't skip breakfast – it's one of the best ways to start your day and fuel your body.

It's also useful to learn to differentiate true hunger from 'emotionally-driven' hunger. Make a conscious effort to start listening to your body – next time you feel hunger pangs, try rating that sensation, from 0 to 10.

Establish 0 for the sensation when you are extremely full up, and 10 for the times when you are very hungry indeed. Aim to tune into your body and learn to gauge your true hunger level. Don't forget that it takes about 20 minutes for the brain to register that you are full up – so slow down.

Ideally, you're aiming to stop eating about 7 (that's the point when you are satisfied but comfortable). When your body is at about a level 3 – in other words when you're able to function but beginning to feel uncomfortably hungry – then it's the right time to eat for true hunger.

Try heeding this rule today. Food will be all the more satisfying when you learn to tap into – and follow – true hunger and satiety.

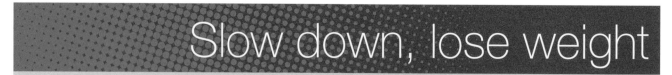

Slow down, lose weight

Eating slowly really can help you lose weight; according to a recent US study, one of the reasons why the French have a history of lower obesity rates compared to Americans is because they spend more time savouring their meals. Eating slowly may help trigger feelings of fullness, explain experts, so you end up eating less. Try:

- Putting your fork down between bites
- Sipping water after each bite
- Chewing your food thoroughly before swallowing
- Using smaller plates (about 9 inches in diameter). Studies also show that people tend to clear their plate when eating, regardless of how many calories this means they consume

Thirst

Many of us often confuse hunger with thirst. Being slightly dehydrated can fool us into craving food – when what we really need are fluids.

The British Dietetic Association recommends that the average 60kg adult should drink 1.5–2 litres (6–8 250ml glasses) of fluids a day – plenty of which should be water. It's good for skin and metabolism and can banish fluid retention.

Aim for about one litre of water for every 1,000 calories of food you consume. Have one glass of water for every alcoholic drink, and for every caffeine-containing drink (such as tea, coffee or cola), have at least half a cup of water to counteract the diuretic effect.

The colour of your urine, though, is the best gauge to assess your hydration levels – you're after a pale watery colour with a tinge of lemon. Yellow urine means you need to drink more.

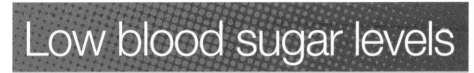

Low blood sugar levels

Not eating enough of the right foods at the right time throughout the day can wreak havoc with your body's blood sugar levels. And when they become out of kilter, you feel tired, drained, suffer low moods – and that's when you experience, and give into, cravings. It's your body's way of asking for a quick energy supply.

The problem is that when our blood sugar levels are low, we're chemically drawn to sweet, sugary foods – the very foods that raise our blood sugar quickly, providing a quick energy burst, but one which is followed by a rapid drop – taking with it your mood and energy.

And so the cycle begins.

The best way to avoid this is to eat little and often – ideally mini-meals based on slow-releasing carbohydrates (see below) with a bit of protein to help fill you up.

Here's a simple low-calorie appetite suppressant: try a snack of hummus on an oatcake or crispbread. The combination of protein and slow-releasing carbohydrate helps rebalance your blood sugar levels and fills you up for longer.

Hormonal triggers: PMS

Research in the Journal of Reproductive Medicine has found that women with PMS are more likely to crave sugary foods, and experts estimate that about 40% of women experience PMS symptoms at any one time – which may include bloating, tiredness and low moods.

Many women also find that they experience cravings for sugary, high-fat foods – chocolate, cakes, biscuits – in the few days before their period.

There may be several explanations for this.

Firstly, there is a metabolic peak in the few days before your period – your body requires a few extra calories a day. Reaching for chocolate – or a similar highly calorific food – may be one way of ensuring the body recoups those extra calories.

Low blood sugar levels (caused when high levels of oestrogen occur) and another possible explanation for the desire for carbohydrates and chocolate in the pre-menstrual days. Basically, your body is after a quick energy boost.

Low levels of serotonin are thought to be another possible explanation for PMS cravings. When your body is producing low levels of serotonin (the mood-enhancing chemical) you're more likely to crave sweet or starchy foods; these kind of foods increase the production of serotonin in the body.

It may be worth swapping your three meals a day for six in the week before your period. Eating regularly means you'll never get too hungry and your blood sugar levels remain stable, so you'll be less likely to munch chocolate.

Also aim to eat plenty of foods rich in vitamin B6; it's thought to relieve the low moods associated with PMS because it helps to raise levels of serotonin. Foods rich in vitamin B6 include lean meat, poultry, fish, eggs, nuts, cereals.

The mineral magnesium and vitamin B6 work well together and are both needed in good supply to make the mood-managing neurotransmitters (chemical messengers) dopamine and serotonin – magnesium-rich foods include fish, green leafy veg, nuts, wheatgerm.

It feels good

There's another good reason why we're drawn to certain yummy foods – again and again. Eating them makes us feel good all over – at least temporarily. Here's how:

When we eat something tasty, the stimulation of our tastebuds causes the release of opioids – the body's own natural version of the mood-enhancing drug morphine.

Foods high in sugar and salt cause the release of higher levels of opioids than other foods – which is why we really like these and crave more of them.

Experts explain that when we eat these foods, the brain sends out chemicals which regulate our appetite – one of which is the hunger-producing chemical neuropeptide Y. In other words, when you eat junk food, foods high in fat, sugar and salt for example, physiological changes take place in the body which mask the hormonal signals that would otherwise tell you to stop eating.

Little wonder some foods are described as moreish. In fact, somewhat controversially, researchers at Princeton University in the US say that the brain changes resulting from high levels of fat and salt are similar to the brain changes caused by heroin.

In their studies, when they fed rats a diet containing 25% sugar, they noticed that the rats became anxious when the sugar was removed, and experienced symptoms similar to the withdrawal symptoms of nicotine or morphine users – chattering teeth and the shakes, for example.

Other studies on rats at the University of Wisconsin Medical School found that when the pleasurable feelings evoked by the brain chemicals that are released eating sweet, salty and fatty foods were replicated using synthetic chemicals, the rats ate up to six times their normal intake of those foods.

The concept that certain foods are indeed 'addictive' is still a hotly debated issue amongst scientists (and women!), but many of us enslaved by a daily salt'n' vinegar or chocolate habit may well agree there's some substance to it

Cravings: what's your poison?

- **Salty foods such as crisps, chips:** it's the taste. Our tastebuds can become so accustomed to salt that foods often taste bland without it.
- **Sugary foods:** sugar is thought to be addictive, and provides the body with a quick energy fix.
- **Cheese/creamy foods:** pleasure chemicals are released in the brain when you eat high-fat foods, which is why you want more of them.
- **Chocolate:** the sugar, fat and pleasurable texture release feel-good chemicals. Chocolate also contains phenylalanine, which is converted by the body into dopamine, a feel-good hormone thought to improve alertness and concentration.
- **Comfort foods/stodge:** high-carbohydrate foods release serotonin – they make you feel full up and leave you with a sense of calm and wellbeing.

Emotional needs

The relationship between mood and food is a complex one. Women are particularly susceptible to cravings triggered by emotions. Experts talk about 'emotional hunger' – that is the desire to eat fuelled not by actual hunger but by boredom, depression, loneliness. It's easy to see how the pattern begins.

Perhaps as a child we were given a chocolate or biscuit to soothe a scraped knee or bump on the head; perhaps good behaviour was 'rewarded' with chocolate and sweets; perhaps Granny cooked our favourite meal or baked us a special cake as a treat; or it may be we were praised for finishing our plate at mealtimes.

In short, many of us from an early age have learned to associate food with love, comfort, nurturing. It's not surprising that those early messages stick, and as an adult, in times of stress, anxiety or loneliness, we reach for the biscuit tin, or treat ourselves to a big plate of our favourite dish.

So how do we start to unpick those early messages? Experts say that recognising your triggers can help you avoid cravings, and by adjusting your habits you can beat your cravings and make sure your healthy eating plan stays on track.

Understand the cycle

1) **The craving trigger:** you've had an argument at work, or perhaps the kids are playing up and you're feeling close to the edge.

- **The craving:** a cup of tea and the contents of the biscuit tin (you can never stop at one…). You feel you deserve a treat at the end of a hard day.
- **The solution:** ask yourself what you're really after. A cuddle? Some sort of physical satisfaction? Try a warm bubbly bath with scented candles – the works, or find other, more nutritious ways to tantalise and satisfy your tastebuds – nibble delicious olives, a bowl of ripe strawberries, artichoke hearts.

2) **The craving trigger:** you're slumped in front of the television, there's nothing much worth watching, you're after a lift.

- **The craving:** something salty and moreish – a packet of Pringles would do it.
- **The solution:** what are you really after? Are your evenings long and dull? could you schedule in a yoga class, or start running with a friend? Make a list of those nagging to-dos – and arrange to do something useful every evening. Could you be more selective about your 'TV nights' – only watch something that really engages you? And prepare healthy TV snacks – a bowl of crunchy crudités with a healthy, low-fat dip, for example.

3) **The craving trigger:** you're feeling down, unmotivated, life's hard – perhaps you're going through a relationship break up or have just lost your job, or are experiencing some other bitter disappointment.

- **The craving:** a large bar of chocolate (or two)… eating something delicious will give you a boost and help you drown your sorrow.
- **The solution:** what are you really after? An answer to the problem you're facing? Some actual human comfort rather than a comfort substitute? Start by finding a shoulder to cry on – sit down with a trusted friend and share your feelings; write it down – putting pen to paper can be very cathartic; take some exercise – vigorous activity helps release feel-good endorphins and leaves you feeling emotionally refreshed. Write down a list of long-forgotten goals – what new project can you take on that will give you a new goal in life? Devise a step by step plan – look ahead, get practical.

Beat the craving 'downward spiral'. Think yourself slimmer and fitter

- Motivate yourself. Write down reasons why you want to beat those cravings. To lose weight? Get fitter and healthier? To handle stress better? To fit into those old clothes? Feel more attractive? It can help spur you on.
- Make your goals realistic and measurable. Devise specific, achievable plans such as losing two pounds each week, or getting in shape for a fun run or family party in two months' time, or ways to control the cravings when they strike. It can help you stay focused.
- Keep your goal in sight; stick a picture of yourself now and at your ideal weight on the fridge, or on your desk at work, as a reminder of what you're hoping to achieve.
- Prepare to celebrate each pound lost or craving controlled as a victory; devise rewards for each goal you reach; treat yourself to a massage, a new outfit, a day at a spa, that mountain bike.
- Remind yourself you're a winner; make a list of other life achievements you're proud of and personal victories. Consult them when your resolve wavers. You can do it.

Stress

Most of us are familiar with this. Working long hours, our constant 24-hour society, a poor work/life balance not only take their toll on our emotional health, they can affect our eating habits too.

When we're stressed, the hormone cortisol is released; cortisol is actually an appetite-booster – it makes you crave sweet foods and carbohydrates which are responsible for the blood-sugar rollercoaster ride.

The hormone cortisol also encourages your body to lay down fat in your abdominal area – which is considered the least healthy place for fat storage. It's vital to have some stress-releasing techniques in place to help you control your stress-induced cravings. Try our relaxation strategies in chapter 6.

24-hour temptation

It's not surprising many of us often become preoccupied with food – and the less healthy variety, too – given the consumer-driven world we live in today. Everywhere we turn we're bombarded by prompts to spend, spend, spend – or eat, eat, eat.

When you're feeling peckish, a billboard or TV advertisement seducing you with delicious goodies is just the kind of trigger that's often too hard to resist. And given the proliferation of TV cookery programmes, it's not surprising that food is always our mind.

From the way products are packaged to the brand image, everything is painstakingly controlled to make foods – chocolate bars, ready meals, takeaways – as attractive as possible.

'Eat this and you'll look ravishing, have more fun, be more successful, happier', the message seems to be.

Supermarkets often make it more difficult to resist junk foods, particularly when they have two for one offers or arrange the store's layout to get our juices flowing.

Children are extremely susceptible to this kind of manipulation, which is why parents are constantly having to contend with pester power.

The best way to overcome temptations is to always write a shopping list – don't impulse buy. Always avoid going to the supermarket when you're hungry. Don't be seduced by cheaper bulk buys. If you buy a packet of six chocolate bars, you'll eat them!

Be selective about your viewing habits – and aim to watch those cookery shows on a full stomach.

SAD

Many people dread the onset of winter – for them it spells months of depression and associated symptoms, including cravings.

According to SADA (the Seasonal Affective Disorder Association), about 500,000 people in the UK are affected by debilitating low moods each winter between September and April, particularly during December, January and February.

It's thought to be caused by an imbalance in the hypothalamus in the brain which happens as a result of the lack of sunlight and shortening of the daylight hours during the winter months.

Natural light is needed to help control our body's natural rhythms of sleep, appetite, mood and energy. But for some people, this lack of sufficient light in the winter months means they are unable to produce sufficient levels of the chemical messengers serotonin and melatonin which govern sleep and mood. As a result, the body's rhythms are out of kilter, and appetite goes haywire.

Carbohydrate cravings are common in SAD sufferers – which have been linked to lower serotonin levels.

Getting as much natural light as you can during the winter can help, and try to stick to slow-releasing carbohydrate-rich foods – brown rice, wholewheat bread and pasta, and other wholegrains such as bulghur wheat, couscous and quinoa.

Regular exercise can help; increasing numbers of studies show it can have a positive effect on mood and body image.

Beat your cravings

So how can you beat the cycle of negative eating and take control of those cravings? Try these techniques:

Eat breakfast

When it comes to boosting brain power, breakfast is the most important meal of the day. Studies have shown that a nutritious breakfast can improve your mental performance, sharpen your concentration and increase creativity. Research also shows that eating a breakfast rich in complex carbohydrates (such as oats, wholemeal) can enhance your memory throughout the morning. In fact, research shows that breakfast eaters tend to make fewer mistakes, work faster and are more verbally fluent than those who skip breakfast.

- Breakfast eaters suffer less from colds and flu, and are reportedly less stressed than people who go to work hungry.
- Eating breakfast is a vital habit to adopt because it kickstarts your metabolism, and provides your body with nutrients as well as energy for fuel.
- For the most nutritious breakfast, focus on slow-releasing carbohydrates. Add a bit of protein (such as yoghurt, milk or egg) and you'll stay fuller for longer. And ideally combine with some fruit or juice, to provide your body with its first dose of disease-fighting antioxidants for the day.
- If you're hoping to shape up as well as sharpen up, breakfast is still a good habit to start.
- One US study found that people who eat breakfast actually eat fewer calories throughout the day than those who skip breakfast, so it can also help you lose weight.
- The body is more efficient at metabolising carbohydrates in the morning than it is in the evening, too, so those calories will be used up by the body during the day rather than being stored as fat as they would be if you ate them in the evening.

Eat protein

Protein helps boost your metabolism, and is a great way to help control cravings because it fills you up. It helps keep your blood sugar levels steady, which means it helps you stay feeling for longer.

Those infamous low-carb diets which were said to help keep Hollywood's A-listers in shape (but also considered nutritionally unsound) may have given protein a bad name, but eating sufficient amounts of the right type of protein can be a vital way to stay slim and keep in control of your eating. (High protein diets come with health warnings from nutritionists as excessive intakes of protein can have adverse effects on your kidneys, bones and breath.)

Experts say about 15–20% of your diet should come from proteins and that we should aim to eat three portions a day. Women need about 45g each day. If you consume a 2,000 calories-per-day diet, roughly 300 of those calories should come from proteins such as turkey, cottage cheese, fish and nuts.

What's a portion of protein?

A portion is about the size of your fist. That's equivalent to an ounce or so of nuts, about 2–3oz (50–75g) cooked lean meat (or a steak that's about the size of a pack of cards), fish or poultry, one egg or 4oz cooked beans.

Here's a guide to how much protein you get in different food sources:			
85g portion lean roast chicken	26g protein	40g cheddar cheese	10g protein
130g grilled cod steak	27g protein	200g tin baked beans	10g protein
boiled egg	8g protein	100g soya beans	14g protein
one pint semi-skimmed milk	19g protein	30g peanuts	7g protein
150g low-fat yoghurt	7g protein	15g sesame seeds	4g protein

Protein facts

Animal proteins such as meat, poultry, fish and dairy produce contain all the eight essential amino acids your body needs, but plant proteins (nuts, pulses, grains and seeds) lack some of these, so vegetarians and vegans should make sure they eat a variety of different protein sources each day.

Here's your guide to proteins and how they nourish the body:

Dairy: yoghurt, milk and cheese are rich in calcium too.

Fish: salmon, tuna, herring, sardines, mackerel, trout are all particularly rich in omega-3 fatty acids.

Beans: a great source of low-fat protein; they're rich in fibre and contain B vitamins.

Nuts and seeds are rich in protein, fibre, minerals, vitamin E.

Seafood, such as prawns, is rich in the antioxidant selenium, vitamin B12 for healthy blood, and iodine for thyroid function, plus they're a tasty low-fat source of protein.

Plain, flavoured or smoked tofu – soya products such as tofu are the only plant-based food equivalent to animal products in terms of protein quality. They're packed with B vitamins, zinc, potassium, magnesium and iron. They're also loaded with fibre and are rich in calcium. Soya products also contain isoflavones which may protect against certain cancers.

Protein tips

- At lunchtime: always eat starch with protein at lunchtime, preferably in the ratio of one portion of starch to one portion of protein; too much starch at lunchtime can make you feel lethargic (as it increases the amount of serotonin in the brain), plus it makes you want to reach for an instant sugar fix sooner afterwards, boosting your calorie intake.
- By balancing your protein and carb portions, you'll fill yourself up for longer, get a better range of nutrients and save yourself calories.
- Try wholemeal pitta with salad, 25g lean back bacon, small boiled egg and sliced tomato.
- Jacket potato with cottage cheese: 200g potato with 150g reduced fat cottage cheese. Serve with side salad.
- Vegetable soup with beans: 500ml carton of non-cream-based vegetable soup with half a cup of kidney beans or quinoa.
- Sushi: mixed medium sushi box (250g). Serve with a small glass of orange juice.
- Open sandwich: 1 slice pumpernickel bread, 100g smoked salmon, 1 tablespoon low-fat yoghurt. Serve with large spinach salad.

Eat Yourself Clever Carol Vorderman

Snack more sensibly

What do you usually snack on? Crisps? Chocolate? Toast? Aim to include protein in your snacks, along with a fruit or veggie. Eating a filling protein means that your snacks will be more satisfying and nutritious, and will stop you eating more later because nothing has quite hit the spot.

Choose from these groups: fruits, veggies, dairy, grains, and meat (which includes fish, eggs, nuts, legumes). So if you fancy a biscuit – just make sure you have it with a glass of milk and an orange too. Burger and chips? Have beans and a fruit salad too.

Be clever with comfort foods

Comfort food doesn't have to mean fat-laden stodge with little nutritional value. It's a question of making lower fat and calorie choices. Here's how:

- Munch warmed fruit loaf with your mug of tea instead of butter-laden crumpets; fruit loaf is rich in fibre and iron and is gooey and moist so you won't need oodles of butter.
- Enjoy piping hot crumbles; they'll keep your fruit intake high. If you swap fat-heavy crumble mixture for brown-breadcrumbs and brown sugar you'll keep it low fat. Serve with (reduced fat) custard and you'll get plenty of calcium.
- Smother your afternoon toast with hummus instead of butter – it's a good source of protein, plus it's high in soluble fibre which lowers cholesterol levels.
- Casseroles and hotpots can be ultra-healthy, especially if you leave them to go cold, then remove any fat on the surface. Stick to lean chicken varieties, or reduce red meat content by adding beans and bulking up your servings. Plus you'll boost your vitamin and mineral intake especially if you add filling root vegetables such as parsnips (lots of vitamin B, C and folate) and turnips (rich in potassium, calcium and vitamin C) instead of dumplings.
- Love roasts? Swap pork for veggies – and use spray olive oils and balsamic vinegar to add taste and cut back on fat.

Choose filling foods

What are the most filling foods, calorie per calorie? According to a study by the Australian researcher Dr Susanne Holt, some carbohydrates curb the appetite more than others. She calls it the satiety index (SI). The key to losing weight is to fill up on low-fat, low-calorie foods. Here's your guide to filling yourself up (these calculations are all based on the same 240 calorie portions):

- potatoes are twice as filling as grain bread
- porridge or oatmeal is twice as filling as muesli
- oranges are almost twice as filling as bananas
- crackers are twice as filling as croissants

Keep busy

People often admit that boredom prompts them to crave salty and sugary snacks. Identify the times of the day when you're most likely to experience cravings – watching the television, for example, or after lunch – and have a few distraction techniques at hand. If you are able to ignore your craving for about 15–20 minutes it may well go away…

- keep your hands busy – take up knitting
- phone a friend
- paint your toenails
- go for a walk
- get online
- clean your teeth

Keep a food diary

Keeping a food diary is an effective way to identify your food triggers and examine your emotional relationship with food. Monitoring everything that passes your lips may also make you more aware of how much you are eating every day. (Experts say we often underestimate how much we eat.)

According a study of dieters published in US journal Health Psychology, those who consistently recorded everything they ate over the festive season still lost weight (about 7lbs over the six-week period between Thanksgiving and New Year), whereas those who didn't keep a record gained about 3lbs.

Start today: write down every thought you have about food, what you ate for each meal or snack. Track those cravings – what prompted them – a thought, emotion, TV ad, genuine hunger? Explore your feelings under temptation. If you gave in to temptation, how did you feel? Understanding your cravings is the first step on the road to conquering them.

Self-monitoring in this way has been found to help people lose weight, and pave the way for a happier relationship with food.

Find other treats

If you can't kick that chocolate or other habit, you need to start thinking laterally. There are ways of giving in to your cravings without piling on pounds or eating large amounts of sugar or saturated fat. Try these healthier treats:

- **Chocolate-covered strawberries:** decadent and delicious, these give you a chocolate 'fix' but a portion of strawberries also provides disease-fighting vitamin C.
- **Toasted nuts in soya sauce:** sprinkle seeds or nuts with soya sauce and heat them in a pan over the hob for a few minutes until they brown.
- **Chocolate Brazils:** a choccy treat, but Brazil nuts are a good source of antioxidant selenium, rich in vitamin E, and contain brain-friendly omega-3 fatty acids.
- **Blueberries with ice cream:** rich in anthocyans known for their disease-fighting qualities, blueberries taste like little sweeties. Combine them with a dollop of ice cream (opt for good quality, ideally organic versions) and you'll get a bit of sugar and fat with calcium too.
- **Big fruit salad with fromage frais:** give rein to your sweet tooth but get a dose of phytochemicals too. Fromage frais provides calcium and a creamy texture without being a high-fat food.
- **Cantaloupe melon:** make believe you're on a desert island. Cantaloupe melon tastes of summer, is juicy and thirst-quenching. It's also a rich source of betacarotene.

Don't ban anything

We all know how depriving ourselves of something can lead to cravings. As soon as you put something on the forbidden list, it becomes the very food you absolutely have to eat.

Feeing guilty when you have succumbed and then banning it all over again just establishes a negative cycle.

Instead, try a more moderate approach. Scheduling treats into your daily or weekly diet has actually been found to help people lose weight and take control of their eating. According to one Canadian study, dieters who were told to give up sweets entirely actually ended up eating more of them than a group of dieters who were told to get 10% of their total calories from sweets. Plus over four months the sweet eaters had lost more weight than those on a sweets-free diet.

The bottom line, say experts, is that if your diet includes a bit of the foods you most like, you're more likely to stick to it. A little of what you fancy....

Try the 10% sweets rule – allow yourself something sweet for each of your meals – such as low-fat mousse, an ice-lolly, a big fruit salad with ice cream, or a handful of sweets for your pudding. (Eat them as part of a meal and you're less likely to have the blood-sugar-rollercoaster effect you experience on an empty stomach.)

It's also worth scheduling the treat into your day – if you know you're allowed a bit of chocolate, you'll look forward to eating it. It will help control your urges. Plus you're more likely to stop at one!

Cognitive Behaviour Therapy (CBT)

CBT has been found to be effective in treating various disorders from mild depression to anxiety, phobias to insomnia to cravings.

It teaches you ways to break the cycle of negative thinking that turns a desire for a food into an overwhelming craving.

CBT involves examining unwanted or unhelpful thoughts, attitudes and core beliefs, and also changing the way in which you behave as a result of those thoughts. It's based on the premise that we often have unhealthy patterns of thinking which lead us to behave in negative ways.

Treatment usually lasts for between 8 and 20 sessions. During the course of the treatment you'll learn techniques to help control your thoughts and change your behaviour, and will be set homework, or asked to read useful books or other material.

Other practical measures include developing coping techniques such as relaxation tricks, e.g. meditations or deep breathing exercises, which may help with panic attacks or anxiety, or help boost confidence. Recent research in the journal Obesity Research found CBT to be more effective in helping control binge eating and curbing overindulgence than medication.

The Department of Health now supports CBT for conditions from depression to bulimia.

Your GP should be able to put you in touch with a number of health professionals who use CBT. For a list of accredited practitioners, contact:

The British Association for Behavioural and Cognitive Psychotherapies (BABCP) www.babcp.com.

UK Council of Psychotherapy (UKCP) www.psychotherapy.org.uk.

Neuro-linguistic Programming (NLP)

This personal development method uses a set of techniques to help you challenge the way you look at the world, and your role within it. It helps you understand that by changing your outlook, the way you behave, or speak or even move, you can improve your attitude and alter negative bad habits such as bingeing.

For more information visit www.anlp.org.

Chapter 4
Smart Foods for Your Table

Certain foods are particularly rich in the nutrients needed for a healthy brain, so it's a good idea to ensure they're on your daily menu and to make a few healthy food swaps where necessary.

The key to a healthy diet is moderation – you need certain vitamins and minerals to facilitate the absorption of other brain-boosting nutrients, so aim to eat regular balanced meals, keep your intake of saturated fats and additives to a minimum, and increase your consumption of fresh fruits and veg.

1) Berries

Blueberries, raspberries, strawberries, blackberries are a very good source of vitamin C and are rich in disease-fighting antioxidants.

They're also a good source of salicylate (which helps fight infection). Plus the skins provide fibre, which is good for your digestive health and can help speed transit time or avoid constipation, which may help keep you feeling more energetic.

Various studies testify to the brain-enhancing powers of berries. Research from the University of Maryland published in the journal Nature concluded that a strawberry-rich diet is an effective way to boost your powers of concentration and thought.

Researchers at Tufts University found that rats who were fed berry extracts showed reduced signs of ageing compared to others.

It's the high antioxidant levels in these fruits which are thought to help protect your cells' DNA and reduce free radical damage – both of which are linked to Alzheimer's disease.

Blackcurrants are one of the richest sources of vitamin C; in fact, one 100g serving supplies you with 200mg of vitamin C, which is five times your daily recommended intake, and also provides you with good amounts of fibre.

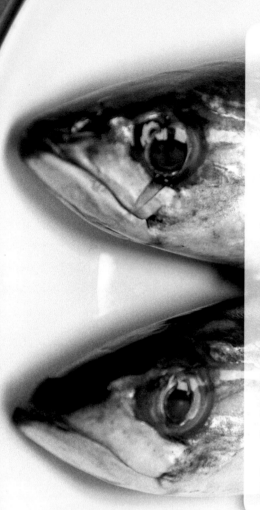

2) Oily fish

Oily fish (such as salmon, pilchards, sardines, mackerel) are rich in omega-3 fatty acids, which are important for brain function. Studies show foods rich in these essential fatty acids can boost alertness and increase concentration.

Your brain is around 60% fat, so a diet rich in essential fatty acids helps keep it well lubricated. Fish oils help strengthen your brain cell membranes and improve brain function by boosting blood flow.

They are particularly beneficial to a foetus's developing brain; pregnant women are encouraged to up their intake of oily fish in the last few months of pregnancy. Breastfeeding mothers, too, are advised to get plenty of fish oils in their diet to maximise their baby's brain development.

Children given healthy amounts of omega-3 fatty acids have been found to do better at school. And ongoing research indicates that symptoms of dyslexia and hyperactivity in children have been helped with supplements of EPA and DHA.

It's thought the DHA in fish oils may help stave off dementia, help memory and alertness, and improve concentration.

Canned sardines which contain bones are also rich in calcium, and if you opt for those in tomato sauce, you also reap the benefits of the disease-fighting antioxidant lycopene.

Sardines and pilchards are amongst the most sustainably caught fish, according to Sustain, the food and farming organisation. Plus these have higher levels of omega 3s than even salmon.

3) Pumpkin seeds

They're tasty and delicious, and make a great snack. Pumpkin seeds are a rich source of vitamin A, potassium and magnesium.

They're a good brain food to have at hand, as they're a good source of the amino acid tyrosine, which your body needs to manufacture the neurotransmitter norepinephrine which you need for concentration, alertness and motivation.

They also contain brain-boosting omega-3 fatty acids. (Linseeds are a particularly rich source of these.)

Seeds can also be a good protein source if eaten in the right food combinations to provide a balance of important amino acids – combined with grains (oats, rice etc) and pulses such as (beans, lentils etc).

Try incorporating them into your everyday meals by sprinkling them on cereals or over yoghurt. They add a lovely healthy crunch to salads, too.

Add them to home-made cakes, breads and buns, and experiment with vegetarian roasts, cutlets and burgers.

Eat Yourself Clever Carol Vorderman

4) Green leafy veg

We would all do well to include several portions of green leafy veg into our daily diet. Our brains would certainly benefit. In fact, studies have shown that eating three or more portions of leafy green veg (such as spinach, kale, lettuce, spring greens) can help slow mental decline by as much as 40%.

It's thought that the rich antioxidants in green leafy veg – carotenoids, flavonoids, and vitamin C – have a protective effect on the cells.

Green leafy veg are also rich in folate, another key brain-protecting nutrient. Folate is believed to help lower levels of the amino acid homocysteine which is thought to increase your risk of stroke and mental decline, as well as heart disease. A study reported in the Annals of Neurology found that increased folate levels and decreased levels of homocysteine in the blood were associated with a better memory.

Plus leafy greens also contain calcium and magnesium which play a key role in nerve transmissions.

Women are advised to make sure to pack plenty of folate-rich foods into their daily diet, particularly during pregnancy or when trying for a baby. That's because folate is particularly important for protecting the foetus against birth defects such as spina bifida.

Research also shows that folate may help alleviate depression (and enhance the body's response to anti-depressants). Folate is also involved in the production of red blood cells and has a role in keeping the immune system working.

It can also help women with abnormal cervical smears; in a study of women on the Pill, abnormal cervical cells gradually decreased in the group that took folic acid supplements.

As folate isn't always well absorbed from foods, pregnant women, or those planning pregnancy, are advised to take a 400mcg supplement. Others are advised to get about 200mcg of folic acid a day.

Folate's great!

Here's how to get your daily folic acid: a 40g serving of fortified breakfast cereal provides about 100mcg; one 80g serving of cooked spinach gives you about 97mcg; one slice honeydew melon contains 50mcg; one glass of orange juice gives you 40mcg; two slices of wholemeal toast with yeast extract add about 120mcg.

5) Eggs

Eggs are a good brain food for all sorts of reasons. Firstly they're a rich source of low-fat protein which your brain needs to build neurotransmitters.

Plus protein-rich foods increase satiety, which means we stay full up for longer. When we're full, our blood sugar levels remain stable, and our concentration and energy stores are not subject to the rollercoaster ride associated with fluctuating blood sugar levels.

Eggs are also a rich source of iron, which is important for providing energy and helping combat fatigue – another key element in mental efficiency. (The iron from eggs is more accessible if you combine it with a vitamin C-rich food or drink – fruit juice with a boiled egg for example.)

Another important nutrient in eggs is choline, which is an amino acid that your body uses to produce the neurotransmitter acetylcholine. Studies have shown that low levels of acetylcholine may impair memory, and are associated with Alzheimer's disease.

Eggs are also a good source of tryptophan, which your body needs to make the neurotransmitter serotonin, important for regulating mood and sleep.

6) Chicken and turkey

A good low-fat source of protein, which is important for physical and mental energy, poultry such as turkey and chicken is rich in minerals such as potassium, iron and zinc. (Dark meat is a richer source of iron than white meat.)

Turkey (and chicken) is a good source of the amino acid tryptophan, which we need to make serotonin. For this reason turkey may be a good food to eat through the winter to help boost levels of serotonin which may be lower in these months.

Poultry is a good source of B vitamins (which we need for a healthy nervous system).

And turkey is a good source of vitamin B12 (chicken doesn't contain so much – although chicken livers are a good source), which plays a vital role in brain health. It's needed for making and maintaining healthy nerve and blood cells, and for making DNA. (Low levels of vitamin B12 are linked to low mood, memory problems and fatigue.)

Poultry contains the amino acid tyrosine which your brain uses to make dopamine and noradrenaline – important for enhancing concentration and mental alertness.

All of which explains why a chicken or turkey sandwich may be an excellent snack when your concentration or energy levels are flagging.

7) Soya

For vegetarians, soya products such as tofu are the only plant-based food equivalent to animal products in terms of protein quality.

They're packed with complex carbs and B vitamins, zinc, potassium, magnesium and iron. They're also loaded with fibre and are rich in calcium.

Recent research has shown that isoflavones, the natural plant oestrogens found in soya foods, may have positive effects on oestrogen receptors in the brain's hippocampus – which could help improve memory. A recent London study found that an isoflavone-rich diet helped improve memory and mental flexibility (the ability to adapt to new situations) in as little twelve weeks.

Good sources of isoflavones include tofu, soya beans and soya milk. Soya products contain magnesium, which works together with vitamin B6 and is thought to help regulate mood.

As a protein source, tofu is low in calories and saturated fat (it contains only 35 calories and less than 2g fat per average 25g serving). Other soya-based products include soya milk, soya beans and soya sausages.

Or try edamame beans. Low in fat, packed with protein and fibre and rich in isoflavones, these trendy Japanese-grown soya beans are sought for their cholesterol-lowering and cancer-fighting properties. They're available in fresh or frozen form.

8) Oats

These grains have been fast gaining a reputation as a great all-round powerfood.

They're a great provider of energy; research at Loughborough University found that porridge may be one of the best foods for short-term and long-term energy boost – studies on athletes found that unsweetened porridge was even more efficient at sustaining them than sports drinks. They're digested slowly which helps keep blood sugar levels on an even keel and provide the brain with a longer lasting supply of energy too. Oats also contain nutrients crucial for healthy nerve health – calcium, potassium, magnesium and B vitamins. They also provide tryptophan which can help boost your mood.

They're also rich in soluble fibre which is important for healthy digestion.

They can also lower cholesterol levels, and protect against cardiovascular disease such as stroke and heart attack.

9) Beans/legumes

Beans and legumes are a good source of protein, although they're best combined with grains such as rice, couscous and bulghur wheat in order to become a more nutritious 'complete' protein. They also provide slow-releasing carbohydrate to fuel the body and brain.

They're rich in fibre too; studies have shown a link between a high-fibre diet and improved cognition.

Lentils are a particularly rich vegetable source of iron, which you need for energy levels, and they also contain small amounts of disease-fighting isoflavones, and are a source of lignans and phytoestrogens. They provide potassium and calcium too – important for healthy nerves.

Red kidney beans are rich in protein. (A 100g portion provides about 16% of a woman's daily protein needs and about 33% of an adult's fibre needs.) They also contain some folate and calcium.

10) Avocados

Avocados are a delicious source of vitamins E and C, whose antioxidant powers can help protect brain health. In fact, one study of 5,000 people reported in the American Journal of Epidemiology found that those with the highest levels of vitamin E in their blood had the sharpest memories.

Avocados are also a good source of the healthy mono-unsaturated fats that can help keep your cholesterol levels low, which helps protect your blood vessels – including those in your brain – and reduce the risk of stroke.

Avocados may have a bad reputation for being a high-fat food, but it's actually saturated fats and trans fats (found in fatty red meat and processed foods, including pastries and cakes) that we should be avoiding.

Your body uses healthy fats such as the mono-unsaturated fats found in avocados to absorb certain nutrients (such as vitamin E), for insulating your nerves and for building cell membranes, so it's a good brain-boosting food.

11) Prunes/figs and other dried fruits

Dried fruits such as raisins, sultanas, dried apricots and figs are rich in fibre and are a good source of instant energy, and also provide iron, potassium and calcium. Figs and apricots contain useful levels of folic acid.

Prunes are nutritious high-fliers, according to experts at Tufts University. They rate extremely highly on the ORAC scale (oxidative radical absorbance capacity), which ranks the antioxidant power of fruits and veg. In fact, their antioxidant power is measured at about 5770 units – way above the minimum of 3500 units we're advised to get in our diet a day.

Prunes are also rich in iron and provide fibre, so they're good for your overall digestive health and can help protect against constipation which can deplete your energy levels.

Sprinkle dried fruit over cereal or fruit salads, plump them in juice for a delicious pudding or compote, or chop up and add to bread or scones.

12) Tea

The good old cuppa is hailed for its health-boosting properties.

Studies show that green tea in particular can help improve your brain health. One study published in the American Journal of Nutrition found that older people who drank two cups of green tea a day were 50% less likely to develop cognitive impairment than people who drank three cups or fewer a week. It's thought the rich antioxidant content of green tea helps stave off mental decline.

But black tea (which is also rich in antioxidants) has benefits too; studies found that its flavonoids inhibit the action of acetylcholinesterase, an enzyme which breaks down acetylcholine, a neurotransmitter which plays a role in memory.

13) Apples

If one a day keeps the doctor away, two or three could keep your brain ticking that bit more efficiently.

That's the conclusion from a study in the Journal of Nutrition which found that apple juice appears to reduce some of the damage to the brain and memory that is caused by free radicals. Other research shows that it may be antioxidant properties in quercetin that give apples their brain-boosting powers. It's thought to help stave off Alzheimer's by protecting your brain's cell membranes. Quercetin is also found in tea and onions.

14) Sweet potatoes

Betacarotene (found in orange-fleshed veg such as sweet potatoes and carrots) is a powerful antioxidant which can help slow down the ageing process, including mental decline, and help fight cancers.

In fact, one humble carrot contains about 6mg of the nutrient, and while there's no official RNI for betacarotene, experts recommend a daily intake of about 10mg.

Sweet potatoes are also a great source of carbohydrate which helps release the good-mood neurotransmitter serotonin.

15) Bananas

Bananas are an important source of potassium (a mineral that plays a role in nerve transmission) and one banana is thought to provide you with as much as 11% of your recommended daily intake. A lack of potassium is linked to confusion and depression.

Potassium can also help regulate the body's salt levels, and can help dilate the blood vessels, helping the blood flow more freely around the body. For this reason bananas are thought to be useful in helping reduce blood pressure, and guarding against heart disease.

Although bananas have a moderate to high GI (which means the sugars are relatively rapidly absorbed by the body), they're still a good source of energy – particularly when you need a quick short burst, such as after exercise when the body needs to replenish its glycogen stores.

Because they're a rich source of carbs, bananas help boost production of serotonin and provide good levels of the stress-busting mineral magnesium.

Bananas make a good snack and topping for cereals and yoghurts, but stick to yellow bananas rather than green ones, which aren't so well absorbed by the small intestine.

16) Wholegrains

Wholegrains such as bulghur wheat, brown rice, wheatgerm, wholewheat pasta and buckwheat (used to make pancakes, bread and pasta) are thought to provide your body with a longer-lasting supply of energy, important for concentration and alertness, than simple, refined carbs. Brown rice is also rich in B vitamins which are needed for cell growth and energy.

The fibre content in wholegrains is thought to help lower cholesterol levels and protect against heart disease.

Try swapping white, refined products for wholegrain varieties; mix your own tabbouleh or Moroccan dishes with couscous. Use wholegrain rice in paellas and with curries; add it to soups or use cold in salad dishes.

(Active men are encouraged to eat 10–11 portions of starchy foods such as grains a day, and active women about 8–10 portions.)

17) Citrus fruits

Citrus fruits are known to be rich in vitamin C, the antioxidant which helps mop up the free radical damage which happens as a result of high levels of stress.

Oranges also contain phytonutrients such as betacarotene, and good levels of folate, which is linked with lower levels of brain decline.

In fact, one average orange contains about 25% of your recommended intake of folate, and almost twice the vitamin C intake.

Dutch studies of people aged 50–70 who took folate supplements showed that those who took daily doses had the mental abilities of those almost five years younger. It helped maintain their ability to process information and reactions involving movement.

18) Nuts

An important smart food, nuts such as Brazils, cashews, hazelnuts and almonds contain various nutrients that can improve your brain function. They're a good source of protein, fibre and minerals such as calcium and zinc, and contain omega-3 fatty acids, good for heart health and brain function.

Hazelnuts and almonds are particularly rich in the antioxidant vitamin E which helps slow cellular ageing; almonds are also one of the richest plant sources of calcium.

Cashew nuts have good levels of the mineral zinc, which is important for immune function and healthy cell membranes.

Nuts are also rich in mono-unsaturated fats which are beneficial for your arteries and blood flow around the body.

Nuts can be quite high in fat and therefore calories so eat in moderation (for example, 100g Brazil nuts contain 682 calories and 68g fat, 100g peanuts 564 calories and 46g fat, and 100g walnuts 688 calories and 69g fat). Chestnuts are lower in fat – only 170 calories and 3g fat per 100g – plus more than 86% of the calories in chestnuts come from carbohydrate rather than fat.

Aim for about an ounce a day – that's about 12 walnuts or 20 almonds.

Toss a handful over breakfast cereal or yoghurt, or add to soup, salads and casseroles. Or try toasted nuts for an easy, nutritious snack.

19) Quinoa

Quinoa is an increasingly popular Peruvian broadleaf plant grain, which is known for its high protein content, vitamin E, calcium and good levels of iron, all of which are needed for the making of neurotransmitters. Plus it's virtually gluten free, so it won't bloat you and is good for those with a gluten intolerance. Its low glycaemic index means quinoa is a filling food, providing you with longer-lasting energy.

20) Broccoli, cauliflower, sprouts

Broccoli justifiably earns its reputation as one of the top smart foods. That's because it's rich in flavonoids which help protect the body's cells from oxidative stress which contributes to disease and ageing (including mental decline).

The cruciferous family (which includes broccoli, cabbage and Brussels sprouts) are rich in calcium, folate and carotenoids, and also provide sulphorane, which has been found to stimulate cell detoxification (and has been linked to reduced risk of breast cancer).

Scientists at Harvard University list Brussels sprouts as one of the top vegetables for lowering your risk of stroke. Stir frying or steaming helps maintain vitamin C levels which are lost when boiled.

21) Mangoes

Juicy and delicious, mangoes contain vitamin C, fibre, betacarotene and potassium, all of which help boost your digestive health and immune system and lower cholesterol.

Mangoes can help boost mental energy levels because they contain vital nutrients (vitamin C and betacarotene) which are known to enhance the body's absorption of iron.

22) Flaxseed oil

Flaxseeds and flaxseed oil provide useful amounts of omega-3 fatty acids and help protect brain cells and their membranes. As these fatty acids are more commonly found in fish, flaxseed products are a good way for vegetarians to access them. Fatty acids can help reduce the risk of heart disease and stroke.

Swap your usual saturated fats or cooking oils for flaxseed, mix for dressings, seasonings and marinades, drizzle over salads. Blend with fresh herbs to make your own flavoured oils. Avoid heating flaxseed oil, though, as the benefits are reduced when heated.

23) Dairy products

Milk, yoghurt and cheese are good sources of energy-giving protein. Dairy products also contain tryptophan which converts to serotonin. Cheese is also rich in tyrosine, which is converted to noradrenaline (which increases mental clarity and alertness). Tyrosine is thought to become depleted when we're stressed, so a yoghurt makes a good snack when under strain.

Calcium is abundant in dairy foods, and it's thought to have soothing benefits, so dairy products make effective good-mood foods.

24) Tomatoes

These are rich in the caretonoid lycopene which has been linked to lower levels of prostate and cervical cancers, and helps keep cells – including those in the brain – better able to fight free radical damage.

Lycopene is best accessed when heated, so tinned, cooked tomatoes are actually a richer source than raw (canned tomatoes provide about three times more lycopene than fresh).

25) Peppers

Red peppers contain the antioxidant nutrients betacarotene and vitamin C, which help fight cancer and heart disease, and slow the ageing process. Red peppers are richer in vitamin C than green ones – one red pepper contains about three times your recommended amount of vitamin C.

Colour your mind

When it comes to getting the most from your fruits and vegetables, think colour.

The deeper the colour, the richer the product is in important disease-fighting nutrients, say experts, and the different colours are indicative of the various phytochemicals in the fruit and veg, so by choosing a colourful spectrum each day, you'll be assured of an assortment of vital health- and brain-boosting nutrients.

According to researchers at Tufts University in Boston, purple/red colours (prunes, raisins, blueberries and blackberries) produce the biggest rise in blood antioxidant levels. When it comes to veggies, think green. Curly kale, spinach and sprouts have the greatest antioxidant capacity out of vegetables.

Also be aware that when it comes to the five-a-day message, five should be your minimum.

How to get your five a day:

- **Improvise.** The good news is that all fruit and veg, whether fresh, frozen, dried or canned, count towards your five a day.
- **Know your portions.** It's about 80g of fruit or veg – which could be about three heaped tablespoons of veg, beans, fruit salad, or a cup of berries/cherries/grapes, a large slice of watermelon, for example, or one pear, apple or orange
- **Drink one.** Even fruit juices count too (although they only count as one portion, however much you drink – aim for a 150ml glass).
- **Don't confuse them.** Potatoes don't count, though (apart from sweet potatoes), but beans (such as kidney beans) and pulses do – but only as one daily portion.
- **Be creative.** Sneak fruit and veggies in where you can: add chopped and diced veg to soups or casseroles, or to sandwiches; add extra veggies to mashed potatoes.
- **Keep counting.** Aim to eat two portions of fruit and veg with each meal, and incorporate other portions into regular snacks so that you're easily clocking up five a day or more.

Think smarter, go Mediterranean

Do you feel relaxed, calmer and possibly sharper on holiday? That healthy Mediterranean diet may be something to do with it.

We know that that the Med diet, which includes smaller portions of red meat, a high consumption of vegetables and herbs, particularly tomatoes, onions and garlic, and olive oil is one of the healthiest in the world.

One new study published in the Annals of Neurology has found that following a Mediterranean diet could reduce your risk of Alzheimer's by as much as 40%.

It's thought the high levels of vitamins C and E, the flavonoids and healthy mono-unsaturated fat can help keep arteries healthy, and thereby keep blood flowing to the brain more steadily.

Plus the nutrients also help fight the free radical damage and inflammation linked with Alzheimer's disease.

How to do it at home:

- **Make sensible but tasty swaps** – ditch margarine for olive oil; choose coarse grain breads instead of white loaves as they're higher in fibre.
- **Treat yourself to a regular glass of red wine** –Zinfandel, Syrah and Cabernet Sauvignon are richer in antioxidants than other varieties. Have drink-free days too, and avoid binge drinking. Don't exceed the recommended limits – one to two each day for women, three to four for men.
- **Vary your diet** – if you eat from the five food groups every day – wholegrain breads and cereals; fruits; vegetables; dairy and dairy-substitute products; and proteins such as meats, nuts, fish, legumes (beans etc) – you could add as much as four years to your life!

Should I go organic?

According to the Soil Association, 30% of our foods have been found to contain residues of chemicals.

One study found that of 4,000 samples of mushrooms, soft fruits and lemons, 90% contained traces of more than one chemical. And apple crops are known to be sprayed with chemicals over 20 times.

Worldwide studies have shown that organic fruits and vegetables contain up to 27% more vitamin C and up to 25% more magnesium than non-organic crops. Salad, vegetables such as spinach, lettuce, cabbage and potatoes, and perishable soft fruits such as strawberries are more likely to be treated with chemicals than other fruits and vegetables.

It's thought that chemicals such as pesticides in food have been linked with cancer, foetal abnormalities, chronic fatigue syndrome, diabetes, and an impaired nervous system.

However, although certain organic fruits and veg have higher levels of some vitamins and minerals such as calcium, chromium and iron, organic produce may be more expensive and that may put people off eating healthy foods.

If the increased cost of making organic choices means you'll end up consuming less fruit and veg, stick to non-organic produce, peel it, wash it thoroughly, but make sure you eat at least the recommended five portions a day.

If you want to be selective about your organic produce, best choices include strawberries, apples, potatoes and leafy salads, as these are often more heavily treated with chemicals.

Chapter 5
Avoid the Brain Drain

Your brain controls how you think, how you feel, how you act and ultimately who you are.

We've seen that without a well-balanced diet your brain cannot work at its best. Eating a diet deficient in key nutrients and overloading on 'junk' food adversely affects memory, concentration and attention span.

You know how you feel when you've been regularly eating junk food, or too often bypassing healthy meals in favour of on-the-hop crisps, chocolate bars and fizzy drinks. Your skin may appear dull, your limbs heavy and lethargic, your mood somehow low. The lack of nutrients (or high volume of 'bad' ingredients) affects every part of your body – and mind.

Junk food is designed to be tasty, moreish, and to be regarded as a treat – one your body and tastebuds want to have again and again and again … But whereas an occasional treat as part of a healthy, balanced diet won't be detrimental to your overall nutrition or brain power, consistent reliance on sugary, salty or additive-laden foods may well be. Almost as important as eating the right foods is avoiding the 'baddies', the brain robbers.

The brain robbers
Junk food

Foods full of unhealthy fats and sugars are bad for our health overall and affect our brain adversely as we'll see below. But the problem is not just that junk food is bad for you (and it is!), it's that it pushes other good foods, essential for brain health, off the menu. Those who survive on processed ready meals and take aways rarely get enough fruit and vegetables, wholegrains and healthy fats that are essential for a well balanced mental state and long-term mental health.

The 'bad' fats

There are two fats that can be bad for your brain, saturated fat and trans fat. For a healthy brain, saturated fat should be limited. However, trans fats are so bad they should be eliminated from your diet as much as possible.

Saturated fat is derived mainly from animal sources – meat and dairy products – and also found in some vegetable oils such as palm. A diet high in saturated fat may be linked to an increased development of Alzheimer's disease: around the world, where communities have a low intake of saturated fat, the incidence of Alzheimer's is lower.

But the real danger from saturated fat is that too much clogs arteries. The brain has a high requirement for blood, to supply nutrients and keep it cool, and it has an extensive blood supply. If one or more of its numerous arteries become clogged, it can lead to 'vascular dementia', a condition where restricted blood flow to the brain affects thinking processes. But that is not the most common danger that too much saturated fat poses for the brain. There's more. A blocked artery in the brain is the cause of stroke, which leads to paralysis, loss of speech and reduced cognitive ability.

Lose the fat without really trying

- Remove visible fat from meat
- Use cooking oil spray for pans – this uses a fraction of the amount when poured into the pan
- Skim fat from stocks or gravies
- Replace oil or fat in sweet recipes with yoghurt or apple sauce
- Swap to semi-skimmed milk and other reduced fat dairy products

However, the fats that really have doctors worried are the trans fats (found in 'hydrogenated' fats and oils, to give them their other name). Trans fats are a relatively new phenomenon. They are a by-product of the food processing industry and result from heating oils and fats to high temperature and letting them cool. This changes the chemical bonds in the fats and turns them into something our brains and bodies have not met in all their long development.

These trans fats are replacing healthy fats in our diets and in our brains. They are taken up directly by the brain and used instead of healthy fats in cells. They do this by getting in the way of the conversion of healthy fats into the building blocks that the brain needs – so they are replacing healthy fats in our brain cells.

If more persuasion is needed, food manufacturers are beginning to remove trans fats from food voluntarily, no doubt looking at the data available and figuring that it is only a matter of time until governments take action But trans fats are still ubiquitous especially in fried and most particularly in deep-fried food. If you are serious about protecting your brain, limit favourite foods such as crisps and French fries to an occasional treat.

It's also worth getting into the regular habit of checking labels. Worst culprits are heavily processed foods such as biscuits, cakes, margarine, pastries, meat pies and other similar products.

The 'bad' sugars

Around a quarter of our total calorie count is needed to keep our large brain working efficiently; we break down food to the sugar glucose, which is our brain's 'fuel of choice'.

Our body has a superlative system for regulating glucose availability. When there is enough glucose in the blood stream for our energy needs (including brain function), the information is registered and the pancreas stops producing insulin, which carries glucose to the cells.

When blood sugar (glucose) falls and more is needed, we get hungry. We eat to supply more sugar (glucose), and this in turn causes a cascade of 'reward' neurotransmitters to be released (dopamine, noradrenaline and adrenaline, for example). These trigger further breakdown of glucose. This in turn causes the release of more insulin from the pancreas. It is an excellent pathway which has worked efficiently for tens of thousands of years.

Ironically, our modern diet, loaded as it is with refined sugar, is rendering us less efficient at this process. Overloading on refined sugar means that we start by producing too much insulin. So our body becomes 'acclimatised' to it – we become insulin resistant. What this does is break the connection between insulin production and hunger. We eat too much and the sugar, not needed by our bodies, is laid down as fat. Insulin resistance eventually results in diabetes, a disease which is rocketing in incidence in the UK and the USA.

What does this mean? One consequence is the epidemic of obesity. Another could be a general lowering of IQ. That sounds dramatic but there is some evidence that refined, sugary foods are bad for your brain. The more sugar you eat, the higher your chances of suffering from mental health problems; refined sugar has been linked to anxiety, hyperactivity and aggression. Most worrying of all, studies have shown that people who eat the most refined carbohydrates (such as cakes, biscuits and sweets) have a lower IQ than those who eat the least. This is not to say that sugar alone makes you stupid – high sugar intake could be linked to other lifestyle choices which are detrimental to your brain – the link needs to be further explored. But without a doubt, refined sugar is bad for your physical and mental health.

Alzheimer's and weight

Being overweight may increase your risk of Alzheimer's disease. Weight gain increases your chance of developing insulin resistance. University of Washington research shows that in people with insulin resistance, there is a 50% rise in brain and spinal cord inflammatory chemicals and beta-amyloid protein, both implicated in Alzheimer's.

Caffeine

In the ancient Traditional Chinese Medicine tradition (TCM), coffee is seen as a strong drug, recommended as a stimulant to be used carefully and treated with the respect that we accord to other strong drugs.

If you want the best for your brain, that's exactly how you should use caffeine – carefully, when you need a boost. Caffeine has been shown to boost performance in IQ tests and improve memory and it is a great temporary lift to alertness and concentration. When you have to stay awake for night driving, grab an espresso.

But the effects are short term. Quaffing large amounts of caffeine on a daily basis makes you less clever, not more clever. (And even the short-term benefits have been questioned by a University of Bristol study: its conclusion was that the improvement in our performance following a caffeine drink in the morning is due to alleviation of the withdrawal effects of doing without our drug overnight, rather than any intrinsic benefits of caffeine.)

Whatever the benefits to the brain of a short, sharp shock of caffeine, there is no doubt that long-term abuse of caffeine is detrimental to the brain in two ways:

- It stresses you out. Caffeine stimulates the adrenal glands which increases adrenaline production and that means more stress. Stress is bad for your brain as we see below.
- It affects the quality of your sleep. For your brain to work optimally it needs enough good quality sleep. Caffeine makes it harder to fall asleep and more likely that your periods of deep sleep will be disturbed. This has a direct effect on your mental abilities the next day.

If you feel very stressed or jittery, and find it hard to concentrate, it might be a very good idea to cut out caffeine from your diet gradually over a period of two weeks and then stay off it completely for a further two weeks. It will be difficult at first, but you may well find the advantages to your mental health worth it. Then the occasional tea or coffee is unlikely to do much harm.

But if you feel that caffeine is not adversely affecting your stress levels or sleep patterns, and want to use it in moderation, you may well be wondering: how much is too much?

Scientists believe that no adverse effects of caffeine are seen in doses of around 240–250mg a day if you stop drinking or eating sources of caffeine about six hours before you sleep (although one study showed that it can still affect sleep up to twelve hours before bedtime, so ideally, you should stop drinking caffeine drinks around lunchtime).

However, a study published in the American Journal of Psychiatry found that those who drank the equivalent of up to five cups of coffee a day (a moderate intake) or over five cups a day (a high intake) had increased levels of anxiety and depression over those who did not drink coffee or had one cup a day. Those who drank the most coffee had the most stress-related illness and the worst intellectual performance. High caffeine intake could be linked to other lifestyle choices that impair the way we think, but given the ubiquity of caffeine in our culture (it's in everything from chocolate to painkillers), it is worth examining your intake carefully and experimenting with cutting down.

CAFFEINE CONTENT – HOW DO YOU MEASURE UP?		
Drink	**Volume**	**Caffeine**
Coffee (filter)	150 ml	110–150mg
Coffee (instant)	150 ml	40–100mg
Coca Cola	150ml	40-50mg
Coffee (espresso, latte or cappuccino)	shot	30–50mg
Tea	150ml	20–100mg
Green tea	150ml	20–30mg
Cocoa	150ml	10mg
Chocolate (dark)	1oz	5–35mg
Decaffeinated coffee	150ml	0.3mg

Additives

Instinctively, we feel that eating foods that appear to consist of a long list of chemicals cannot be good for us. However, those additives with E numbers have been checked for safety – that's what the E number means. That said, there has been pressure on food manufacturers to reduce the number of additives in foods, especially those aimed at children, and some have complied. Food additives have been linked with behavioural problems in children but there is no generally accepted evidence that the additives still available in food are making our children's behaviour any worse.

However, common sense tells us that overloading our bodies (and brains) with chemicals that they would never meet in nature could be taking a risk with health. Even if additives are not directly affecting our brains adversely, then they could be getting in the way of vital minerals and vitamins needed for a well balanced mental state. For instance, one study showed that the additive tartrazine (E102) 'neutralised' the essential mineral zinc so that it wasn't available to the body. The researchers believed that this might be linked to emotional and behavioural differences in children who consumed tartrazine, although this is not yet proven.

The point is that we do not really know what effect these thousands of additives in modern food will have on our long-term health. But the signs are that it may not be good news and it makes sense to limit them as much as possible. Choose fresh juices rather than fizzy drinks; start looking at labels.

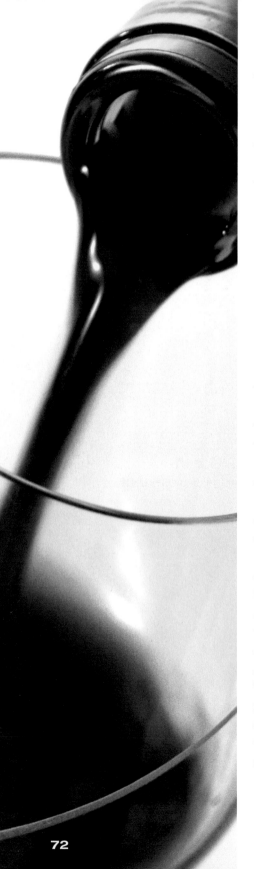

Alcohol

Like caffeine, alcohol can be beneficial to the brain in small amounts. In a study of 500 people with family risk factors for Alzheimer's, those who had one or two drinks per week scored 6% higher at word list recall than those who abstained. Why? We're not entirely sure, but a moderate amount of alcohol may relax us sufficiently to have beneficial effects on the brain. (Stress is not good for the brain as we will see below.)

But as soon as the amount of alcohol you consume rises above a very moderate level, you risk damaging your brain. Even a little alcohol affects perception – which is why drinking and driving is against the law. Drink too much and alcohol impedes the conversion of the essential fats that the brain needs. Memory begins to suffer. Eventually this leads to the cognitive impairment that we all know is a side effect of drinking too much. In a nutshell, drinking too much over a period of time will make you stupid.

Alcohol is also a powerful depressant. A little alcohol makes you convivial but this is probably a function of lifting inhibitions. Too much alcohol affects neurotransmitters' function (notably serotonin) and this makes those who drink to excess gloomier and more stressed.

Too much alcohol is toxic to the brain, but that, of course, does not mean that the occasional glass of wine is going to do you any harm. Your liver is working hard to neutralise the effects of alcohol so that the effects are not felt in your brain. As a rule of thumb, a healthy liver can handle around one unit of alcohol an hour. Drinking moderately at this sort of rate means that you are unlikely to be damaging your brain. Put very simply, avoid getting drunk. Being drunk means that your liver is not able to process alcohol as fast as you are drinking it.

The binge-drinking culture especially amongst teenagers may be particularly dangerous. The British government has followed the example of the French and US governments in recommending that pregnant women don't drink alcohol in case they damage their developing babies' brains. There seems little doubt that heavy drinking harms brain development. In one study at the University of California – San Diego 34 teenagers were given a memory test. Those with alcohol problems showed more activity on brain scans than non-drinkers. Which sounds good, except that, by the time the children had grown up and gone to college, the scenario had reversed. College students who had drunk since their teens scored lower. Young teenage brains may over-compensate for the damage done by alcohol (hence those good results) but eventually, the researchers think, the damage might be too much to overcome.

Eat Yourself Clever Carol Vorderman

Salt

The brain needs small amounts of salt to function optimally; sodium chloride, to give salt its proper name, is needed to keep body fluids at the right levels, to help transmit electrical impulses around the body and brain, and to help cells take up nutrients.

However, too much salt causes the body to hold on to water, which causes the volume of bodily fluids to increase.

Consuming too much salt has been linked to coronary heart disease and hypertension. And large volumes of fluid circulating in the brain put pressure on the brain's blood vessels, increasing your risk of stroke. Hypertension (also known as high blood pressure) causes symptoms such as headaches, sleepiness and confusion.

- Aim to start watching your salt intake; experts recommend we have no more than 6g of salt a day (or 2.4g sodium).
- Cut back on processed foods, which contain lots of salt. Limit your consumption of cured meat and hard cheese. When possible make your own stock, sauces and soups; processed versions are salt-laden.
- Aim to drink plenty of fluids every day (at least eight glasses) and eat potassium-rich fruit and veg (such as bananas, leafy vegetables); potassium helps balance fluid levels.
- Swap salt for fresh herbs, spices, lemon or mustard to flavour your food instead.
- Cook from scratch – apparently 70% of our salt intake comes from processed or pre-prepared foods.
- Get salt savvy – as a rule, foods that contain more than 0.5g of sodium per 100g serving (or 1.25g of salt or more per 100g) are high in salt. Foods that contain less than 0.1g sodium (0.25g salt per 100g) are considered low-sodium foods.
- Start looking at the labels to assess the salt content of packaged foods. Some products only label sodium content, not salt content. To work out your salt intake multiply the sodium figure by 2.5 to find the amount of salt. So if there's 0.6g sodium in 100g and you're eating 300g of it, you're getting 4.5g salt. (0.6 x 3 = 1.8g sodium. 1.8g sodium x 2.5 = 4.5g salt)

Clean up your act

One way to examine the effects of a bad diet is to look at cultures where the population don't indulge in these foods. The Okinawan people live on a 'necklace' of islands between Japan and Taiwan. They do not eat processed food, smoke or drink alcohol or caffeine. Instead they have a diet high in fish, seafood and vegetables. An Okinawan has four times more chance of celebrating their 100th birthday than a Briton: they are the most long-lived nation on earth.

Smoking

Smoking is terrible for your health. Naturally, it is bad for your brain, too. It has been estimated that there are 400 miles of capillaries (tiny blood vessels) in the human brain. This huge network is needed to keep the brain cool and to take a constant supply of oxygen and nutrients that is needed to keep your brain firing and fizzing with ideas. As we all know, smoking causes furring of blood vessels. This limits the nutrients reaching your brain but even more sinister is the chance of brain damage.

Just as smoking can increase your chance of a heart attack by damaging blood vessels that serve your heart, it can increase your chance of stroke by damaging the blood vessels of your brain. So it's not surprising that studies show that half of all smokers who do not give up will die from their habit.

If you smoke, the single most important action you can take to improve your long-term health is to give up.

The good news is that stopping smoking immediately normalises the decline in lung function. So if you give up at 30, your lifetime risk of dying from smoking-related diseases is almost the same as that of a never-smoker.

New research shows that you're almost four times more likely to give up if you go to an NHS smokers' clinic than if you try going cold turkey alone. The drug Zyban and nicotine patches are useful too. If you smoke, give up as soon as possible. See your GP about Smoking Cessation programmes.

Trying to give up? Have healthy snacks on hand to nibble – sticks of celery, grapes or blueberries; it gives you something to do with your hands, and provides powerful antioxidants which counteract the free radicals caused by all that smoking.

Stress

You have probably heard of the term 'good stress'. This refers to the kind of stress that gets our heart racing and fuels our motivation to excel at that important presentation or shine at the party where the person we're really interested in is sure to overhear our conversation. Good stress gives us an 'edge' so that we think quickly and appear alert and intelligent.

But living with constant stress has quite a different effect on our mind. Constantly bathing our brain in the stress hormone cortisol makes us frazzled and liable to error. Just two weeks of stress can cause damage to the brain cells, and Yale University research shows that memory centres are damaged in people who suffer from post-traumatic stress disorder. It's thought that stress makes it impossible for us to lay down short-term memories – which is why we forget important things when we're really up against it!

Stress is bad for your brain but what is so pernicious is the way that it creeps up on us. Take a long hard look at your life and ask yourself if stress could be contributing to forgetfulness, depression or anxiety. If so, it is time to reclaim your life for yourself.

We'll explore useful ways to relax and beat stress in the following chapter.

Water and the brain

Dehydration can slow your brain. The Mayo Institute in the US says dehydration is a major cause of physical and mental tiredness. Being aware of this is particularly important as we get older because research shows that as we age, our sense of thirst is less reliable. Remember to drink even when you don't feel you need to. A good tip is to have a glass with each meal, and after every trip to the loo.

Dehydration is a major cause of mental tiredness, so remember to drink plenty of water.

6 weeks to a better brain

It's much easier to replace bad habits with good ones if you take little steps. Each week incorporate a new good habit (and keep the ones from the weeks before) and in just six weeks you will have made over your health for the better.

Week 1	Drink a large glass of water with every meal
Week 2	Swap one of your regular cups of tea or coffee for a cup of green tea (four cups a day are linked to reduced risk of Alzheimer's)
Week 3	Eat one piece of fruit at every meal
Week 4	Alternate a glass of water with every alcoholic drink
Week 5	Eat at least one vegetable at every meal
Week 6	Take five minutes in every hour to relax no matter how busy you are

Read on to discover which good habits are worth adopting if you want to boost your brain power.

Chapter 6
Healthy Brain Habits

Good nutrition is vital in helping delay mental decline and keeping your brain in its best shape possible. But it's just one part of the picture; there are other factors that play an important role, too. Here's how adopting some healthy lifestyle habits can have a significant effect on your cognitive function.

Get enough sleep

If you've ever had to concentrate hard, or perform at your best the day after a poor night's rest, you'll know all too well how important sleep is for the brain. Most of us agree we feel lacklustre, lethargic and down in the dumps after a bad night, and would admit that a series of late nights or disturbed sleep can damage our physical, mental and emotional wellbeing. Sufficient sleep helps maintain healthy brain cells and plays a role in regulating your mood and sharpening concentration.

As you pass through the stages of sleep, your body's growth hormone is produced which helps all your cells repair and regenerate. Sleep enables our mind to process the day's events and activities (dreams often facilitate this), to repair and heal the body.

- Getting a good night's sleep can boost memory, and help newly formed memories and skills get organised in the brain.
- Experts tell us lack of sleep affects our immune system, too, and makes us more susceptible to infections.
- Skimping on sleep can also cause weight gain. When you're tired, your willpower is weakened, so you're more likely to reach for fatty, sugary or salty foods, and skip that exercise session.
- Research also shows that women who get fewer than five hours' sleep each night are one-third as likely to get diabetes. One reason may be because the lack of sleep may reduce levels of the hormone that tells you to stop eating.
- Insufficient sleep can interfere with hormone production. Some studies have shown that losing just 1.5 hours' sleep for one night can reduce your alertness in the daytime by as much as 32%.
- Another study showed that people who went to bed six hours later than their normal bedtime performed as badly in attentiveness and reactions as those who were legally drunk!
- Sleep deprivation is linked to accidents such as Chernobyl and the Challenger shuttle explosion, and thousands of accidents take place every year as a result of tiredness.
- Fatigue is often blamed for relationship strife, parenting problems, ineffectiveness and discontent in the workplace. One study of sleep deprivation showed that a fifth of sleep-deprived people said they were dissatisfied with life, and over 10% said they felt angry.
- Even short bouts of sleep deprivation raise blood pressure, pump extra stress hormones into your bloodstream and raise blood sugar levels.

Are you getting enough sleep?

Research shows that the optimum amount of shuteye tends to be somewhere between 6.5 and 8.5 hours a night. Japanese research shows that you'll live longer if you get 6.5 hours to 7.5 hours' sleep.

Most people, about two-thirds of us, sleep between 6.5 and 8.5 hours each night. But less than 20% of us get less than 6.5 hours' shuteye.

So how much is enough for you? Sleep experts say the best gauge is to ask yourself if you're waking up each morning feeling refreshed. Are you able to function at your best? If so you're probably getting enough.

Try keeping a sleep diary to assess how you're feeling each day. If you need a stiff coffee to liven you up, then you may need more sleep, and could do well to improve sleep hygiene.

What's keeping you up?

Hormonal fluctuations during puberty, pregnancy or peri-menopause (transition to menopause) can cause sleep disruption as can PMS.

Plus, as you age, you're more likely to experience conditions that interfere with a normal night's rest, such as sleep apnoea (repeated blocking of the airwaves at night) and restless leg syndrome.

Too many stimulants such as caffeine (also found in colas, tea and chocolate) and alcohol may disrupt your natural sleep patterns.

Nicotine is a powerful stimulant and can trigger adrenaline, which revs you up. Studies show smokers tend, on average, to take twice as long to drop off as non-smokers, and sleep about half an hour less.

People with a sedentary lifestyle may be more at risk of sleep problems than regular exercisers.

And of course emotional problems such as stress and anxiety are major causes of insomnia. Stress hormones deplete the feel-good hormones serotonin, melatonin and GABA (gamma-amino-butyric acid) so it's little wonder prolonged stress keeps you up at night.

Depression is often linked to insomnia, and prolonged lack of sleep can lead to depressive feelings.

And hands up all those who regularly engage in late night over-activity, such as computer games or watching stimulating films into the wee hours: anything other than sex at bedtime can conspire to keep you awake.

Some experts also believe that exercising late at night can mean you take longer to nod off, so the best advice may be to schedule your fitness activity for earlier in the day.

Sleep well, stay slim

If you ever find yourself heading for the fridge or, worse, the cake tin when you're feeling tired, you're certainly not alone. Many people find that skimping on sleep is one of the biggest triggers for over-eating. There are reasons for this.

Firstly, it makes sense that your willpower may be weakened when you're sleep deprived – and if it's sheer willpower that is leading you to the healthy section in the supermarket, and away from the junk foods, then without it many of us are on a slippery slope!

What's more, research in the journal Revue Neurologique has found that sleep loss can disrupt your physiological rhythms. When your body becomes unbalanced in this way, you may experience hunger or a desire for fuel at other times of the day – which could lead to overeating. Lack of sleep and out-of-kilter physiological rhythms may also deplete your energy levels. That may mean you simply find you're too tired to exercise – and, as we know, exercise can be an effective appetite regulator, as well as a good way to utilise excess calories.

And another study published in the Journal of Endocrinology and Metabolism found that when you experience lack of sleep, your body's supply of the hormone leptin drops. Leptin helps regulate appetite and metabolism, and when it's in shorter supply, you're likely to eat more. By getting sufficient sleep, you'll stay in better control of your appetite and be more able to master your cravings.

Get more sleep: your good night guide

Rethink your bedroom décor; aim for a clear, cool, uncluttered bedroom decorated in muted colours

- To get a better night's sleep try an early-morning stroll (it can help the production of melatonin which helps regular sleep).
- Get up at the same time even at weekends, take a warm bath at bedtime, and exercise for 30–45 minutes during the day.
- Wind down with music; studies show that listening to soft music 45 minutes before bed for three weeks can improve your sleep by 35%.
- Try yoga; one US study found that a 20-minute yoga session at bedtime helps reduce insomnia; patients fell asleep longer and slept longer.
- Massage may help; research published in the International Journal of Neuroscience found that when people with low back pain were massaged regularly they slept better than patients using other forms of treatment.
- Stop worrying; make a list of all the things you have to do the following day. Keep the list by your bedside and add entries as they occur to you. This way you'll be prepared for the challenges ahead.

Eat Yourself Clever Carol Vorderman

- Meditate: close your eyes and try to empty your mind of daily worries. Slow your breathing, and repeat a particular word or sound to yourself, such as 'peace' or 'calm' or 'sleep'.
- Move your body; people who exercise tend to sleep better than sedentary people.
- Go Eastern; practising Tai chi three times a week for six months has been found to help people sleep longer and more soundly.
- Lose weight; overweight people are prone to sleep apnoea, and snoring, which can disrupt sleep. Keep your weight down by taking three to five half-hour sessions of exercise each week, and watching what you eat.
- Finally, sex in the evening is great for getting a good night's sleep.

Improve your sleep hygiene
The London Sleep Centre recommends the follow golden rules:

1	**Stick to a regular bedtime and wake-up schedule** Aim to go to bed and get up the same time each night and morning. Don't go to bed too early or you may have trouble falling asleep, or your sleep may be restless.
2	**Cut back on naps** Napping can disrupt normal sleep cycles. Try skipping your nap and see if regular sleep patterns improve.
3	**Make your bedroom a 'quiet room'** Don't watch television in your bedroom. Keep your bedroom for sleep and sex only.
4	**Establish relaxing before-bed routines** Have a bath or a glass of warm milk, or do some light reading before bedtime.
5	**Develop relaxation techniques** Try yoga, deep breathing or quiet meditation or listen to soft music while trying to fall asleep.
6	**Avoid troubling news right before bed** Violence in newspapers or on television may bother some people and make it difficult to sleep. Try reading a book instead.
7	**Avoid stimulants** Don't have drinks containing caffeine (tea, coffee, cola) six hours before bedtime. And avoid alcohol or tobacco; they may calm you at first, but they can disrupt your sleep during the night.
8	**Exercise regularly** It helps the body and mind stay healthy, but avoid vigorous exercise right before bedtime.

Eat for better sleep

- Tryptophan-rich foods can help ease anxiety, promote sleep and boost morning alertness. Sources include bananas, dairy foods, nuts, eggs, soybeans, tuna, turkey, cottage cheese, baked beans and chicken. Keep the serving size small and have your snack about an hour before bed.
- Don't eat late: it raises your body temperature and keeps your body and brain switched on. Eat early evening – a couple of hours before bedtime. That way your metabolism will drop (which is conducive to sleep).
- Cut out caffeine and alcoholic drinks within 4–6 hours of bedtime. Alcohol reduces the amount of time you spend in deeper stages of sleep. Instead stick to camomile, lemon balm and passion-fruit tea.
- Eat for sleep: avoid cruciferous veggies such as cauliflower, cabbage and broccoli in the evening if you're prone to bloating as they can make you too uncomfortable to sleep.
- A carbohydrate-rich meal at the end of the day can help you feel relaxed and sleep better – try a risotto or pasta dish, or even a bowl of milky porridge. Avoid fatty, meaty or creamy meals as they're harder for your system to digest.
- Avoid sugary foods late at night; they can raise your blood sugar levels, which gives you a burst of energy.
- Magnesium-rich foods have been found to help fight depression and low moods and encourage sleep. They include green leafy veg, nuts and wholegrain cereals.

Prepare the bedroom

Leave the window open; the optimum bedroom is well ventilated and completely dark (so invest in blackout curtains in summer). The best temperature for sleep is 'cool' – about 60–65°F (16–18°C), cold enough to require a blanket.

Top tip:Burning the candle?

If you have a vital presentation or exams to study for, and need to put extra hours in, sleep experts say you're better off working later rather than geting up earlier in the morning. Studies show sleeping in the early morning between 2am and 6am is more restful and beneficial than late night sleep (between 10pm and 2am).

Tryptophan–rich foods such as bananas can help promote sleep

Exercise

Exercise and your brain

Given that your body reaps noticeable benefits when you exercise, it makes sense that your mind does too. There's a wealth of evidence to show the link between exercise and brain and mood.

One recent study from the Journal of Gerontology found that exercise triggers a measurable growth of brain volume in older people; in three months, exercisers had the brain volume of people three years younger.

Other research found that even three 15-minute sessions of exercise a week can help protect you from dementia later in life.

There are various reasons for this. Firstly, exercise is thought to help boost cerebral blood flow and stimulate the growth of new cells in the brain. What's more, staying active can help keep you slim, which is another important key to keeping your brain in good condition; research has found that obesity is linked to a decline in mental ability over the years. Researchers think this is linked to the hormone leptin which is secreted by stored fat – it's thought high leptin levels may affect learning and memory. The link between obesity and memory decline doesn't just affect older people; even young thirty-somethings with high BMIs are thoughts to be at risk of accelerated mental decline.

There are all sorts of other benefits of taking regular exercise, too – it helps elevate mood, boosts your metabolism, can alleviate PMS and period pain, and can reduce your risk of heart disease.

Exercise to music – and boost your brain!

A recent study showed that listening to music while you're exercising can boost your brain power. People who listened to music during physical activity did better on a verbal fluency test than people who exercised without music.

How much, how often?

Experts recommend three 20-minute sessions of vigorous activity per week (where you become out of breath), or five weekly 30-minute sessions of moderate activity (such as a gentle walk).

The good news is that one study from Loughborough University found that three 10-minute sessions of exercise produce the same beneficial results as one tougher 30-minute session – and can be easier to fit into your day.

Exercise and mood

Depression is widespread; according to statistics, we all have a 1 in 5 chance of suffering from depression at any one time, and women are twice as likely as men to suffer.

However, taking steps to keep in control of stress and anxiety levels and developing coping mechanisms can reduce anyone's risk. Exercise can be a powerful mood regulator.

Studies show that regular exercise can reduce your risk of depression and anxiety; one study in the journal Health Psychology found that 30 minutes a day – broken up into 10-minute sections – was enough to improve mood and regulate emotions. That's because feel-good endorphins are released during periods of vigorous activity.

Exercising outdoors has additional benefits – studies show being in the open air surrounded by greenery has mood-boosting effects too.

A dance-based class is a good idea too; anything set to music with an upbeat tempo will give you a boost.

Exercise to calm the brain

If your brain is on overload, a workout could be just what you need. One study in the Journal of Behaviour Research and Therapy showed that regular exercise helped reduce people's sensitivity to anxiety.

Tai chi and yoga are known for their relaxing benefits. But fitness experts say that high-intensity workouts (try running, uphill cycling etc) show more pronounced and lasting effects in reducing stress levels than low-intensity exercise, possibly because you release more endorphins during intense workouts.

Alternatively, repetitive exercise such as treadmill running or swimming laps is great for a stressed mind. It doesn't require any mental input and can help you feel calm.

Moving your body – even when you're feeling lacklustre – is actually a great way to fight fatigue; one new study from the American College of Sports Medicine found that regular exercise boosted energy levels and decreased fatigue in about ten weeks.

A gentle low-intensity exercise such as yoga or Pilates may actually make you feel more energised. One study showed that yoga was more refreshing than even taking a nap.

Tai chi is a gentle martial arts discipline which combines slow, gentle, flowing movements with controlled breathing. Studies show that it can help offset cognitive decline, stimulate brain-eye co-ordination and improve body aware-ness. Apparently, stroke victims who practised Tai chi found a significant improvement in recovery.

Prepare for action: getting started

If you're new to exercise, or are not sure where to start, or can't always find the motivation to put on your trainers, these 'go get it' tips may help:

- Make a list of your reasons for wanting to get fit – pin them up somewhere, or carry them around with you to keep you focused.
- Make sure you start with an activity you actually enjoy – if running's not for you, try walking, cycling, swimming, try martial arts or learn flamenco.
- It may help to schedule your exercise sessions into your week – writing them into your diary as you would a doctor's appointment.
- It's also worth teaming up with an exercise buddy; studies show working out with someone else can be more motivating than exercising alone.
- Beginners or those who've reached a fitness plateau may benefit from a session with a personal trainer. Just one can help you set goals, assess your fitness levels, take you on to the next stage.
- Aim to schedule your exercise sessions in the morning; research found that you're more likely to stick to it if you workout before midday.
- Splash out on the right gear, too; you may find you'll get in the right mood and perform better if you're wearing quality trainers or sports kit.
- Give yourself a specific goal – such as a charity fun run or five-a-side friendly. It can help keep you motivated.

Relax

We all know that stress and anxiety can cloud our mind and prevent us from firing on all cylinders. There's no denying we feel mentally fresher, sharper, more focused and more productive when we're calm and relaxed. Our brain's 'creative juices' can flow more freely when we're unfettered by worries.

That said, stress is an inevitable part of modern life. Studies show that as a nation we're less happy than we were in the fifties, despite the fact that we're three times richer. Recent research found that only 36% of us would describe ourselves as 'very happy', and one poll found that four out of ten of us think life has become worse in recent years.

Stress clearly plays a part in all this discontent. We're working harder – longer hours – than ever. According to the International Stress Management Association, nearly a third of us are finding it stressful balancing work and home lives.

What's worse, according to the British Heart Foundation, half a million people in the UK believe that work stress may actually be making them ill. Nearly 70% of us complain that we don't have enough time to ourselves – and the downside of chronic stress is the ill-effect it can have on our health, relationships and general wellbeing.

That's not to say that a bit of stress isn't helpful. That old 'fight or flight' response that our ancestors experienced in the face of man-eating predators was appropriate – helpful. It's true that even now many people find that the adrenaline rush from working on a tight deadline, or before a presentation can give them the edge and spur them on to great things.

However, problems arise when the work life balance becomes out of kilter, or when life is too stressful to cope with. Many of us are under so much pressure today. But the truth is, living as we do in a 24-hour society can take its toll on our health and emotional wellbeing if we don't keep it in check.

Stressing out: what's happening in there?

When we're under stress, our body goes into the 'fight or flight' response. Our breathing becomes shallow and rapid, the heart beats faster, our blood pressure rises and stress hormones cortisol, adrenaline and noradrenaline are released, which slows down digestion.

Blood sugar levels also rise to provide the body with instant energy. Stress can lead to poor eating habits (such as reliance on junk food), and other unhealthy behaviours such as excessive drinking or poor sleeping habits, which can also rob your brain of the vital elements it needs to work most efficiently.

Persistent and prolonged stress has been linked to ailments from muscle tension and headaches to cancer and heart disease, as well as mental disorders. It has also been found to compromise the immune system.

Putting a stop to stress

The key, then, is to ensure we set aside time to relax, de-stress and spend time with those we love. Any activity that we find relaxing may have the potential to boost our immune system because it counteracts the stress response – by lowering blood pressure, decreasing pulse rate, regulating your heart rate and reducing damaging stress hormones in the body.

So how do we learn to relax, stay positive and find happiness? Start by identifying your stress triggers. Ask yourself what is stopping you from being happy right now. Financial worries? A relationship crisis? Too much work? Not enough time to look after yourself?

Once you've identified the root causes of your stress, you're better able to start tackling it and find lasting solutions.

Relaxation techniques for everyday calm

- **Chill:** aim to spend at least ten minutes or so alone in the peace and quiet. Perhaps put pen to paper and plan how to make small adjustments to your life to lower your stress levels.
- **Change your thinking:** try to view issues or problems in a different light; working on changing your perspective can turn mountains into molehills. Make a list of the all the things in life you have to feel grateful for now.
- **Get closer:** one survey showed that nearly 48% of us believe that relationships are the biggest factor in making us happy, and yet one in 25 of us speak to no friends at all in an average week. Setting aside time to be with your friends or your partner is important; research shows that a long-term, loving relationship can make you as much as 6.5 years younger.
- **Sniff some therapy:** Bach Rescue Remedies are flower essences which are thought to help rebalance your emotions and overcome negative feelings. You pop them on your tongue or take two drops diluted in water in moments of need – whether that's before a stressful meeting at work, or when you're having a stressful day with the children. Try sweet chestnut when your outlook's bleak or gentian if you're feeling despondent.
- **Get some Bs:** intense stress depletes the body of vital B vitamins which are important for everything from the nervous system to a healthy heart to releasing energy. Take a daily supplement. Also aim to get plenty of vitamin B foods in your diet, including lean meat, green leafy veg and wholegrains. Foods rich in tryptophan (fish, chicken, avocados, cottage cheese) are said to have calming effects on the body and can help stabilise mood.

- **Listen to some music:** relaxing to music has been found to help stabilise blood pressure, heart rate and levels of stress hormone cortisol. Classical is often best, say experts; research in the British Journal of Health Psychology shows that listening to classical music helps lower the blood pressure after a stressful task.
- **Release the anger:** instead of repressing them, try writing down your feelings – penning a letter to anyone to whom you feel angry or resentful can be cathartic. In your letter explain how you feel. Vent all those feelings you're keeping inside. Imagine yourself purged of the anger and pain. Make sure you sign off your letter on a positive note, though. Perhaps explain how you coped or what you've learned from the experience. Then destroy the letter.
- **Pamper yourself:** book yourself a massage: research shows it can help fight pain and slows down the release of cortisol. Or wallow in an aromatherapy bath: essential oils are known for their rebalancing qualities. Try bergamot (uplifting and relaxing), clary sage (soothing, rebalancing), cypress (a tonic), lavender (restorative and relaxing), ylang ylang (balancing, comforting).
- **Visualise a detoxified you:** sit or lie on the floor breathing deeply, in for a count of four, then out to a count of four. Imagine your whole body suffused in a clean and re-energising white light. Imagine it streaming slowly through the top of your head. As it cascades down, imagine the stresses and strains of life and negative thoughts being washed away. deep breathing helps you keep your equilibrium.
- **Go green:** Take a walk in the country or the park; surround yourself with greenery. A study in the American Journal of Preventive Medicine says it can help you stay healthy and less stressed.
- **Watch a funny film:** laughing triggers the production of dopamine which induces euphoria; it's said to stimulate the same part of the brain as drugs such as cocaine!
- **Try colour therapy:** pale blue and green are considered restful colours. Or surround yourself with splashes of pink; it's uplifting, and restorative. Research conducted by the Prison Service and London's South Bank University in a project to reduce incidence of suicide and self-harm in prisons found that pink had a calming effect on prisoners.
- **Create your 'quiet place':** no space, no problem. Close your eyes and imagine a beautiful, tranquil sanctuary – a beach, forest, beautifully furnished or cosy room. You're creating a private escape from the world, a place of comfort and serenity. Make it yours. In times of stress, conjure it up again and escape to your imaginary safe haven.
- **Eat for relaxation:** aim to include good amounts of magnesium-rich foods in your diet – important to help boost mood. Green leafy veg, nuts and wholegrain cereals are good sources. And avocados, bananas and tomatoes also contain serotonin, which can help regulate your mood.
- **Treat yourself:** simple pleasures such as a glass of wine in the garden may have a protective effect on your mental health because, quite simply, doing things that make you happy is going to help keep you happy.
- **Yoga:** the carefully controlled deep breathing helps invoke calm, and adopting postures can relieve stress and tension in muscles. A study in the Journal of Alternative Therapies in Health & Medicine found that people with mild depression reported a decrease in anxiety and improvements in mood following a one-hour class of yoga each week.

Chew your way to a sharper mind

Schoolteachers have always had a zero-tolerance approach to chewing gum – chewing it in the classroom was always a no-no – but perhaps they should think again. There is evidence that chewing gum may help boost brain activity, and improve your concentration levels and alertness.

One study by Japanese researchers in 2001 found that chewing gum increases blood flow to the brain by as much as 40%.

It's a link backed up by another more recent study, published in the journal Appetite, which found that students who chewed chewing gum while doing memory tests experienced an increased long-term and short-term memory by 35%.

Studies conducted by the University of Northumbria in Newcastle and the Cognitive Research Unit in Reading asked 75 adults to undergo various memory and attention tests which involved words and pictures and the ability to remember telephone numbers. One third of the group was asked to chew for 20 minutes, another third was asked to mimic the chewing action, and the rest didn't chew at all. Some of the groups chewed during the learning part of the test, and chewed again when asked to recall the word list. Others chewed only at the learning stage of the test and not during the recall part.

What the researchers found was that those who chewed during the test – and then again when asked to recall the words – performed better by as much as 36% in some of the tests. Those who chewed when learning the words, but didn't chew the gum during the recall part of the test, didn't perform quite as well.

The researchers found that the heart rate of the chewers was faster than the non-chewers. The theory is that chewing raises the heart rate which causes more oxygen and nutrients to be pumped around the brain. The researchers didn't attribute the results to any ingredient in the gum itself, but to the effect of blood flow boosting memory.

The scanning equipment used in the test found that brain activity in the hippocampus increases when people chew, but returns to normal when you finish chewing. So if you want to perform well – get chewing!

Mint condition

Sniff your way to a brighter brain. Studies have found that the scent of peppermint can make you more alert and increase your powers of accuracy. Keep some essential oil of peppermint on a tissue in your desk or in your handbag.

Try ginkgo biloba

This herb, originally found in China (and thought to be the world's oldest living tree), has been impressing the scientific world for decades.

It's thought to be good for boosting memory, concentration and other brain functions, and improving blood circulation to all parts of the body, and is considered particularly useful for people with dementia.

It comes from the leaves of the ginkgo tree, and has been used by the Chinese for thousands of years.

Its impressive results are believed to be due to powerful antioxidants called flavoglycosides, which have been found in studies to have neuroprotective effects on spinal cord injuries in animals.

Ginkgo also contains substances called terpene lactones which are known to improve blood flow and reduce inflammation; in fact, one German study shows that ginkgo biloba increases blood flow around the body by as much as 57%.

Studies on ginkgo and dementia have found that it's effective in slowing mental deterioration. And a recent Cochrane report review in association with the Alzheimer's Society found that participants taking ginkgo showed improvement in mood and emotional function as well as cognition. The researchers concluded that there is 'promising evidence of improvement and cognitive function associated with Ginkgo'.

Ginkgo's far-reaching benefits include impressive results with the neurological disease multiple sclerosis. One study at the Oregon Health & Science University School of Medicine's Department of Neurology found that ginkgo may improve concentration in MS patients with cognitive impairment; patients in the study who took ginkgo biloba performed better in tests measuring attention and sorting information, and showed quicker responses in planning and decision making.

Another study published in the journal Nature Neuroscience found that people with Down's Syndrome may be able to boost their memory by taking a supplement.

Studies certainly offer evidence that this herb may be an effective brain booster, at least for dementia. There are several brands of herbal supplements available at chemists and healthfood shops, but check with your GP before taking, in case of contra-indications with other medicines.

Research has shown a link between a high-fibre diet and improved cognition. Try beans, or wholemeal toast with Marmite for breakfast.

Meditation

Sitting still for a few minutes a day, breathing deeply and slowly as you focus on a single object, or word, is like giving your brain a rest.

In fact, various studies have found that meditation can help decrease blood pressure, lower your heart rate and boost blood flow.

Recent research found that it may stimulate the growth of brain tissue and reduce cognitive decline associated with ageing; a small study found that people who were long-term practitioners of meditation experienced an increase in the thickness of the parts of the brain involved in attention span and sensory perception.

People who meditate every day have been found to experience improvements in mood and lower stress levels. Plus research published in Neuroreport found that meditation may stimulate growth of brain tissue.

Sounds like a useful long-term habit to adopt.

Other research has found that people who have practised meditation for many years have increased gamma brain wave activity; gamma waves represent brain activity involved in attention, memory and learning.

Another study found a link between meditation and immune function; it's thought that stress suppresses the immune system, so there may be a stronger immune response in people who find meditation relaxing.

There's also research to show that meditation can help regulate blood pressure; patients being treated with medication for chronic high blood pressure found that two 20-minute sessions of transcendental meditation (TM) each day helped reduce blood pressure, according to a study in the American Journal of Hypertension.

So how does it work? Transcendental meditation involves focusing on a phrase or mantra and allowing thoughts to float in and out of the mind without focusing on them.

Give it a try. There are many CDs and cassettes available, or try joining a class.

Here's how to try it at home. Try sitting quietly for 10–20 minutes a day, breathing slowly, focusing on an object, clearing other thoughts from your mind. When other thoughts come into your mind, try to bring your thoughts back to your original focus.

Brain booster

Find your nearest maze. Some experts say that navigating your way through a maze is a great way to boost your brain power and sharpen your faculties because it exercises both hemispheres of your brain at the same time.

Eat Yourself Clever Carol Vorderman

Use it or lose it

Another important strategy for keeping your grey matter healthy is to exercise it constantly.

Crossword puzzles and other challenging pursuits are thought to strengthen connections between nerve cells, and maybe even help form new neurons.

Learning a language can also give your brain some exercise, as can reading and doing sudoku.

In fact, experts have calculated that regular mental stimulation via exercises such as crosswords and sudoku can keep your brain up to 14 years younger.

Sharpen your mental alertness
Try these brain teasers:

- Think of 20 words beginning with B within 30 seconds
- Within 30 seconds find an opposite for each of the following words: massive, weak, next, failure, fat, happy, lively, critical, open, clumsy
- Within 60 seconds find a word that means the same as each of the following words: Chatty, finish, book, clean, ship, wealth, argue, obscurity, habit
- Read the following eight words out loud twice: sun, vitamin, table, orange, pencil, horse, fruit, joy. Now close your eyes and say the alphabet backwards, then try to remember the words in the correct order.

Keep your brain guessing: breaking the brain's routines helps release neurotrophins which enhance your mental fitness and could boost creativity. Try writing or brushing your teeth with your non-dominant hand. Or get in the car, close your eyes and try to put the key in the ignition.

Chapter 7
Children and Families

As parents or carers of young children, it's important we realise that the 'house rules' and lifestyle habits we establish early in life have a powerful impact on a child's brain.

What you give your child to eat, and the sleep and lifestyle habits you encourage them to adopt, can do great things – or detrimental ones – to their mental agility. So what can you do to boost the brain power of even the youngest member of your family?

In general, the same rules that apply to adults apply to children, too. In fact a healthy, balanced, nutritious diet and regular exercise are even more crucial to a toddler's young body and brain, or a growing ten-year-old with a busy school life and extra curricular activities to balance, or a teenager about to embark on important exams.

When you consider the link between mood and food you can see how getting the right nutrients – whilst avoiding the wrong foods such as junk and additives – and staying fit may have a powerful effect on behaviour, which in turn can affect family life, your child's learning ability and their developing relationships.

Children and nutrition

Here's a good guide to follow when planning your weekly menus. Bear in mind that top nutritionists recommend that each day children should have:

5 portions of fruit and veg
4-6 portions of grains and potatoes
2 portions of protein-rich foods
2 portions of calcium-rich foods and
1 portion of healthy fats (olive oil, fish, avocado etc).

The under 2s should have full fat dairy products – their growing body and brain need the fats.

It's also important to steer your child away from additives. One government-funded study at the UK's Asthma and Allergy Research Centre found that certain food colours and preservatives are linked to hyperactive behaviour in as many as one in four young children. They recommend that all children would benefit from the removal of artificial food colourings from their diet. Avoid fizzy drinks, and limit sugary, processed foods to a minimum.

Incorporate fish or fish oils into your child's diet (aim for two portions of oily fish a week – salmon, mackerel, herring or sardines). Recent Durham Sure Start trials, assessing the effects of fish oil supplements on pre-school children, found that children's concentration dramatically improved after taking the oils. The omega-3 fatty acids in fish oils are thoughts to have a positive action on the brain's neural transmitters. Researchers and parents noticed the children's concentration improving within a week of taking the supplements. Omega-3 fatty acids are also being studied for their positive effects on hyperactivity and dyslexia.

It's also important to ensure your child has sufficient amounts of iron in his or her diet. Iron deficiencies have been linked with delayed development and behaviour problems in young children. Good sources include red meat, leafy green veg, legumes such as beans, and wholegrain bread. Research has shown that children deficient in iron have lower IQ levels than children with sufficient intakes of iron, who also performed better on comprehension tests.

Children should also get plenty of B vitamins in their diet – these nutrients help release energy from food and fuel the growing process. Good sources include brown bread, cereal, Marmite, eggs and oily fish.

A healthy intake of calcium is another crucial nutrient for good health into adulthood – most of the calcium in the adult skeleton is formed between the ages of 8 and 17. Good sources include dairy products and fish.

Eating breakfast is a vital habit to instil in children, as it provides a good supply of energy levels needed for a challenging day at school. Porridge is an ideal choice as oats are especially good for providing mental and physical stamina, and stabilising blood sugar levels which ensure longer lasting energy.

Hydration levels also impact on your child's cognitive function. Make sure your child drinks plenty of water – it's vital for energy levels and concentration. One study at an Edinburgh school found improved test results amongst children who drank plenty of water. When children are dehydrated they'll get tired and their ability to focus and concentrate may suffer. Aim for four to six glasses a day.

Although it's harder to control a teenager's eating habits than it is your pre-schooler's, it's important they understand the importance of a healthy diet. Bear in mind that many teenagers are low in certain minerals such as potassium, magnesium, zinc and iron. See chapter 2 for good sources of these nutrients.

It may also be worth talking to your pharmacist or GP about supplementing your child's diet with a good multivitamin.

Establish healthy sleeping habits

Sleep is such an important factor in maintaining mood and energy, but many children burn the candle at both ends or get into poor bedtime habits, which impair their performance at school. The effects of lack of sleep may be unmistakeable in a screaming two-year-old, but insufficient shuteye can also take its toll on older children.

The first rule for parents is to make sure your child's bedroom is conducive to sleep. If possible, keep televisions and computers out of the bedroom. Stick to natural fibres, invest in black-out curtains to keep the room dark, and establish regular bedtime and wake-up habits – and be strict about them. Avoid serving heavy meals late at night, or try offering a warm milky drink or story to encourage your child to relax. Many areas offer sleep clinics where parents can go to discuss with experts any sleep problems their children may have – talk to your GP.

Teenagers naturally sleep later than younger children. However, early nights and regular habits are still important. Follow these Sleeping Tips for Teenagers from The Sleep Council (www.sleepcouncil.com / 0845 058 4595):

- Try to impress on your teenager the importance of sleep and the need for at least eight hours' sleep on school nights
- Encourage regular exercise – 20 minutes three times a week will help
- Suggest a reduction of caffeine intake (in coke drinks as well as coffee)
- Point out that eating too much or too little close to bedtime – having an over-full or empty stomach – may prevent sleep onset, or cause discomfort throughout the night
- Try and get your teenager into a going-to-bed routine – suggest that doing the same things in the same order before going to sleep can help
- Ensure a good sleep environment – a room that is dark, cool, quiet, safe and comfortable
- Make sure your teenager has a comfortable bed. It may be time to get a new one – and encourage him or her to choose it themselves
- Don't give teenagers hand-me-down bedding. A good rule of thumb is, if the bed's no longer good for its first user then it's not good enough for a teenage child either

Eyes: gateway to the brain?

One study by the City University Department of Optometry and Visual Science found that 12 per cent of children have undetected visual problems, and that a further 43 per cent have never had an eye examination, so don't delay in getting your child tested.

Poor eyesight can cause headaches and dizziness and may be linked to impaired concentration or lowered performance at school.

Under the NHS, every child under 16 (and everyone under 18 in full time education) is entitled to a free eye test, and parents are entitled to a voucher towards the cost of any glasses or contact lenses prescribed for their child. See your GP if you suspect your child has eye problems, or see your optometrist about a free eye test.

Weight and teenage girls

If there's one issue guaranteed to preoccupy a young girl's mind (other than boys) it's weight. Incidence of eating disorders is increasing, and girls are subjected by the media and Hollywood to constant reference to the hallowed size 0 as the 'ideal'. Thousands of teenage girls are constantly 'on a diet', and, as a result, falling well short of the nutritional requirements that ensure healthy development and optimum mental energy.

While worries about underweight girls and those with eating disorders are one side of the coin, the other is the increasing incidence of obesity among children and adolescents.

Not surprisingly, then, puberty is a challenging time for many teenage girls.

Studies have shown that women are at risk of putting on weight during puberty when the surge in the hormone oestrogen causes fat stores to increase to give you female contours and curves.

Research has shown a link between early menstruation (starting your periods younger than 12) and obesity in later life. But experts explain that this may be because overweight girls have greater fat stores, which can be a trigger for menstruation.

According to the World Health Organisation, after puberty both boys and girls develop an increased taste for fat in their diet; but in girls the taste is greater.

Plus teenage girls often avoid exercise by trying to get out of games at school, and are more likely to go on and off faddy diets which can play havoc with their metabolism.

Many parents are too busy to cook regular meals for their kids these days. And the array of fast food and sugary snacks on offer can fool teenagers into eating more calories than their bodies need.

What's important is to avoid the pitfall of the fad diet. What can you do to make sure your teenager stays healthy and well nourished?

- **Encourage her to take more exercise** – dance, skating or jazzercise may be more appealing than netball.
- **Skip the bus and walk or cycle to school.**
- **Make sure you cook an evening meal** – and aim to sit down to eat as a family as often as possible.
- **Teach teenagers to cook** – remind them that it can be a very seductive skill (look at Nigella Lawson) and a good way to learn about healthy eating (rather than obsessive calorie counting).
- **Limit the time spent on a computer** – sedentary lifestyles are linked to obesity.

Student nutrition

When they fly the nest and start university, there's little you can do to ensure they're getting a healthy diet. And many students find they gain pounds during the first months or years away from home in further education as a result of poor nutrition.

In fact over in the US, weight gain in the first year of college is known as the Freshman 15 because the prevailing myth is that students can gain up to 15lb in the first year of college. Recent studies show that both men and women are likely to gain weight during their student years – from about 3 to 10lb in the first two years.

Factors to blame are the endless sitting round in coffee bars, the constant boozing, or the fact that new students often have less structured mealtimes, do more grazing on high-calorie snacks, drink more, are less active and have to watch the pennies without having the experience of budgeting for meals and planning menus.

The trouble is, the same elements that cause weight gain – inactivity, poor nutrition, junk food – are also those that impede brain power, just at the time in life when it's so important.

It's hard for parents to intervene from afar – all we can do, perhaps, is give some advice, lend them our cookbooks and send healthy food parcels!

Brain tips for students:

- **Cook regular meals** – team up with friends, pool your resources, start a rota
- **Opt for healthier snacks** – fruit, crackers, and nuts and seeds (these are good for brain power)
- **Keep an eye on late-night eating** – instead of high-calorie pizzas and kebabs when the student bar closes, try cheese on toast, boiled eggs or stir fries
- **Increase the amount of starchy foods in the day** – bread, pasta, potatoes and noodles are relatively cheap and provide energy

Men and women: different nutrition needs

We know too well that carrying surplus pounds can dent your mood, make you less inclined to exercise and affect your mental and physical energy.

But did you know that your man may be to blame (isn't he always!)?

The truth is, studies have found that women gain weight when they move in with – or live with – a man.

One study of the eating habits of women in the UK and in the Netherlands found that living with a man is one of the biggest factors leading to obesity in women. Another study showed that newlyweds gain on average six to eight pounds over a two-year period after getting married.

So why does this happen? For a start, it's thought that women often end up eating bigger, man-size portions and that couples tend to indulge in more 'treat' luxury foods when they're living together.

Perhaps you're more likely to share several bottles of wine a week, spend cosy nights in with a high-calorie takeaway, and become less active as you spend more time at home together.

Also bear in mind that men often have different food choices – they prefer to binge on savoury foods like pies, steaks and chips. So if you keep him company, in time there'll be more of you for him to love.

What's more, many women may also admit that they relax their fitness and healthy eating when they're no longer under pressure to look for a partner!

Think about your family eating habits – do you serve foods your husband/partner favours? Do you eat similar portions? Have those occasional treat takeaways become more regular occurrences? Have you swapped the treadmill for TV dinners à deux these days?

There's plenty you can do to address the issue:

- **Rethink portion size** – men need 20 per cent more calories a day than women – serve up accordingly. Use a smaller plate for yourself if it helps you reduce your servings.
- **Make a resolution to declare treat foods 'treats' again** – that means you eat them just once a week, or indulge in one big Sunday blowout rather than a huge slap up meal every night of the week.
- **Limit the alcohol** – stick to a glass of wine a night or a pricier bottle once or twice a week.
- **If he likes his 'man food', try to make healthy versions** – make pies with sweet potato topping instead of pastry, or roasts without the fatty gravy, served with big portions of vegetables.
- **From now on ban eating in front of the telly, and make a pact to get active** – why not take up a sport you can do together?

Exercise – get everyone moving

Regular exercise ensures there is plenty of blood pumping round the body – delivering important nutrients to your organs, including your brain. Staying active also gives you energy and vitality and helps keep you sharper and brighter. The benefits of physical activity to children are far-reaching:

- It helps reduce your risk of certain diseases
- It's good for self-esteem and mental wellbeing
- Active children are also less likely to become smokers
- Practising a sport or activity teaches kids countless extra skills from co-ordination to concentration

Unfortunately, it's thought that only three out of ten boys and four out of ten girls are meeting the recommended hour a day of physical activity.

The problem is, the National Curriculum only allows for two hours of sport a week. What's more, a study in the Lancet showed that kids need closer to 90 minutes of exercise each day to ward off heart disease and obesity.

So why aren't our kids moving enough? It's thought that increased hours spent in front of the television or computers may be to blame, alongside the fact that most children are driven to school these days instead of walking.

The challenge for many parents, then, is to get their kids motivated and off the couch.

Here's how:

- Experts say the key is to make sport sociable. Teenagers in particular are more likely to participate if their friends are involved too. Take a group of girls to the tennis club or swimming pool. Plan expeditions and make it a sociable outing rather than 'sport'; team up with other families and go mountain biking or walking. Try rounders or games of frisbee in the park, or skittles with family versus family. Suggest dancing, ice skating or jazz funk style classes for girls, or trampolining.
- Take the boring factor out of 'exercise' and instead find a hobby you can do as a family – try sailing, wall climbing, or windsurfing holidays. Horse riding and even paintballing involve getting active!
- Lead by example. Experts maintain that children of active parents are more likely to become active themselves. Keep it fun and be enthusiastic about sport and exercise.
- Catch 'em young – sowing the seeds early helps. If you can get your toddlers and pre-schoolers active regularly, it will be a normal part of their lifestyle.
- Give kids a sense of achievement – set goals such as beating their previous score, or keep a chart of their achievements. Swimming or running clubs, fitness centres, local races and competitions all help give your child a focus and something to aim for.
- Bribe them… hey, whatever works! Why not promise rewards for each goal achieved – stars or stickers, new trainers or kit for older kids?
- Tap into their celebrity obsession – does their latest pin-up go surfing? Kickboxing? Or do Pilates? Encouraging your child to follow suit may work wonders.

Boost the family's brain power

Experts say that parents who interact and play with their children are giving them a great start in life and helping to stimulate their young brains. So switch off the television and plan some brain-boosting family activities today.

- Instead of disappearing to different parts of the house, plan family events – such as games nights or competitions. Team up with other families or neighbours and organise competitions. Play Scrabble or Trivial Pursuit, or make up your own pub quizzes (minus the alcohol).
- Take them to a maze – navigating your way through a maze is thought to be a great way to exercise grey matter (as well as their legs).
- Limit the time spent in front of the television and computers. Some experts say 1–2 hours a day is enough, and that the under 2s shouldn't watch any at all. Schedule TV- and computer-free nights – and be strict about them.
- Play memory games. 'I went to market and I bought…' – where you remember each person's purchase and then add your own – is great fun and a good brain exercise for little ones.
- Encourage a love of music. Some experts say that having music lessons may increase IQ by a few points. Listen to classical music together or try taking them to a classical concert.
- Expand their horizons. Swap the usual days out at a theme park with visits to the local museum, art galleries or National Trust properties. Most offer children's activities too.
- Have a cards night. It gets them thinking and can help boost their memory.
- Be a bookish family. Getting your children into the habit of reading from an early age is more likely to foster a long-lasting love of books.
- Get Dad involved. Research shows that children of fathers who are involved in their upbringing – taking them on outings, playing together and playing a role in their education – tend to perform better at school than children of more 'absent' fathers.

Bigger babies, better brains?

According to researchers from the Centre for Urban Epidemiologic Studies in New York, babies who are a little bigger at birth often show great intelligence later in childhood. Researchers studied 3,484 babies born between 1959 and 1966. They also tested brothers and sisters so that they could separate the effects of birthweight alone from the effects of different diets or other factors.

The babies' birthweights varied from 3lb 5oz (1.5kg) to just over 8lb 13oz (4kg). Seven years later they tested their IQ. They found that in general, higher birthweights were associated with slightly higher IQ – the average difference between babies of less than 2.5kg (5lb 8oz) and those of up to 4kg (8lb 13oz) was 10 IQ points.

Other studies have revealed similar results – research in Denmark found that birthweight increases correlated with increasing IQ until the baby reached 4.2kg (9.24lb). Although it's yet to be proven, it is thought the relation between birthweight and size comes down to better nourishment in utero during vital stages of brain development.

Eat Yourself Clever Carol Vorderman

Chapter 8
28-Day Eating Plan and Recipes

The following 28-day brain-boosting eating programme is based on meals which combine nutrient-rich fresh fruit and veg to nourish and protect the brain's cells, and low-fat protein served with slow-releasing carbohydrates to give you a long-lasting supply of energy to help boost concentration.

- Aim to eat at least five daily portions of fruit and veg to fill you up and help beat cravings. Smoothies, soups and salads are good ways to increase your daily intake.
- Swap white bread, cakes, biscuits and sugary breakfast cereals for oats, wholegrains, brown rice and wholewheat pasta, rye, pumpernickel, bulghur wheat, sweet potatoes. Slow-releasing carbohydrates (those with a low GI) help regulate your blood sugar levels. They provide longer-lasting energy, and help fill you up.
- Make sure you eat protein at each meal – and include protein in some of your snacks, too. Keep your consumption of fatty red meat to a minimum; choose lean cuts. Good proteins to boost brain power include fish, eggs, lean meat, legumes, nuts and seeds, tofu and dairy products.
- Drinking plenty of water helps boost the absorption of vitamins and minerals, keeps you hydrated (dehydration depletes energy levels) and can increase concentration. Ideally drink 6–8 glasses a day.
- Make fish a part of your weekly diet; ideally aim for the two portions a week recommended by government health experts (one of these should be oily fish). However, because some oily fish contain dioxins and pollutants, we're advised to follow safe maximum consumption levels (see below).
- Aim to ensure your alcohol consumption stays within recommended limits (14 units for women, 21 for men). It will help you stay clear headed and sleep better.

Safe levels of oily fish

Young children, pregnant, breastfeeding women or women intending to become pregnant should not eat more than two portions of oily fish each week. Pregnant women can eat up to four medium cans of tinned tuna. (Fresh tuna is considered an oily fish.) There's no limit on canned tuna for other women. Men can eat up to four portions of oily fish each week, and there is no limit on tinned tuna. (That's because the canning process reduces some of the dioxin content.)

How to eat yourself clever

In this four-week plan you'll find a selection of recipes for nutritious and delicious breakfasts, lunches and dinners, plus healthy snacks to keep you going through the day.

Follow the day-by-day programme, or mix and match the meals and recipes to create your own plan. Within four weeks you should be feeling brighter and sharper, and may even have even have lost excess pounds, which may help alleviate physical and mental lethargy.

Cooking Methods
The way you cook your food has a huge impact on its nutritional value. Here's how to get the most out of food:

- **Keep the nutrients.** Steam instead of boiling. Boiling can damage water-soluble vitamins such as vitamins C and B, so wherever possible, steam vegetables. Some experts believe steaming helps retain as much as 70 per cent of their vitamin C. If you must boil, use as little water as possible, and serve your veg al dente. Keep skins on foods when possible – in many fruits and veg large amounts of nutrients are contained in the skin. And cutting veg in large chunks helps retain nutrients. Roasting vegetables at high temperatures helps seal in maximum amounts of nutrients.

- **Lose the fat.** Grill or griddle instead of frying. Frying coats your food with unnecessary levels of fat (and calories). Grilling and griddling allow the fat to drip away from the food. Don't forget you can steam chicken or fish too. Or try them lightly poached, or in casse of fish seared – but always make sure chicken and pork are fully cooked. When sautéing choose unsaturated fats such as olive, sunflower or rapeseed oil instead of butter or lard (saturated fats). A hand spray is a good way of minimising surplus fat – lightly coat the pan. When cooking meat and fish, you'll retain more of the vitamin B that leaks out into the liquid or drippings if you use it as soup or sauce. Make sure it's not fatty though!

- **Raw vs cooked.** Eating more salads and raw fresh fruit boosts your vitamin intake. Plus their higher water content means they have more filling power – so you're less likely to binge on high-calorie processed food. Raw food needs more chewing so, again, helps fill you up and regulate your appetite. However, some antioxidants – lycopene and betacarotene – are made more available by cooking. So although you're better off eating most vitamin C-rich fruit and veg – oranges, strawberries, red peppers, blackberries – uncooked, you'll get better antioxidant benefits by eating carrots, spinach and tomatoes cooked.

Week 1

Day 1
Breakfast: Seeded Granola with Maple Syrup, Coconut and Dried Fruit (see recipe page 110)
Glass fresh orange juice
Lunch: Hummus on rye bread, with mixed watercress, avocado and tomato salad
Fresh fruit, e.g. kiwi fruit, strawberries, blueberries
Dinner: Cumin Spiced Chicken with Roasted Butternut Squash and Broccoli (see recipe page 128) served with couscous
Snacks: Handful mixed nuts and raisins
Fruit yoghurt

Drinking orange juice with your iron-rich cereal means your body absorbs more vitamin C.

Day 2
Breakfast: Melon and Peach Smoothie (see recipe page 142)
Boiled egg on pumpernickel toast
Lunch: Pasta with Hazelnut and Basil Pesto (see recipe page 134)
Bowl strawberries and natural yoghurt
Dinner: Grilled Sardines with Sicilian Flavours (see recipe page 124) served with new potatoes
Handful grapes
Snacks: Small bag apricots
Fresh fruit

Why not sprinkle some seeds or nuts over your fresh fruit? You'll absorb more vitamin E if you eat fresh fruit with a fat source.

Day 3
Breakfast: Low-fat natural yoghurt with granola, apple puree and handful mixed nuts
Glass fresh orange juice
Lunch: Puy Lentil Soup with Pumpkin and Fennel (see recipe page 117)
Dinner: Baked Sweet Potato with Feta, Chilli, Coriander and Toasted Pumpkin Seeds (see recipe page 133)
Snacks: Oat Banana Pecan Muffin (see recipe page 109)
Fresh fruit

Swap regular baked potatoes for baked sweet potatoes and you'll get lots more betacarotene.

Include plenty of folic acid rich foods in your diet – leafy green veg and peas – as they help your body absorb iron from foods.

Day 4

Breakfast: Banana and Blueberry Smoothie (see recipe page 142)

Slice wholemeal toast with Marmite, cup of herbal tea

Lunch: Pitta filled with chicken and mixed green salad leaves

Fromage frais

Dinner: Filo Parcels with Salmon and Feta (see recipe page 119) with new potatoes

Snacks: Peanut butter on rye toast

Bowl raspberries

Swap refined breakfast cereals for porridge and you'll feel fuller for longer.

Day 5

Breakfast: Porridge with skimmed milk sprinkled with seeds and raisins

Cup of tea or herbal/green tea

Lunch: Stir-fried mixed vegetables (broccoli, green beans, beansprouts, courgettes etc) served with cashews and on a bed of rice noodles

Apple

Dinner: Haddock Wrapped in Bacon, with Anchovy, Rosemary and Lemon (see recipe page 120) with a baked potato

Snacks: Avocado drizzled with olive oil, black pepper

Bowl blueberries

Swap coffee for green tea or juice. Large amounts of coffee can reduce absorption of B vitamins.

Day 6

Breakfast: Pot of plain or soya yoghurt served with teaspoonful of Manuka honey and fresh fruit

Lunch: Sweet Pea and Avocado Soup (see recipe page 116)

Served with slice wholemeal bread and hummus

Dinner: Roasted Soy Chicken with Sesame Seeds (see recipe page 127)

Strawberries in Red Wine (see recipe page 141) served with brown rice

Snacks: Small bag dried apricots

Two rice cakes with peanut butter

Eat your salads with a bit of healthy fat – it helps you absorb more disease-fighting antioxidants.

Day 7

Breakfast: Muesli sprinkled with spoonful berries and handful of mixed nuts

Lunch: Tuna Nicoise Salad (see recipe page 138)

Pot fruit yoghurt or fromage frais

Dinner: Cumin Spiced Chicken with Roasted Butternut Squash and Broccoli (see recipe page 128) served on Basmati rice

Snacks: Sesame Yoghurt Dip (see recipe page 114) served with mixed crudités (chopped celery, carrots etc)

Piece fresh fruit

Week 2

Day 8

Breakfast: Porridge with diced, dried apricots, semi-skimmed milk
Glass orange juice
Lunch: Quinoa and Basmati Pilaff with Dill and Roasted Tomatoes (see recipe page 131)
Dinner: Stir-fried chicken or tofu with Asian greens on a plate of soba noodles
Fruit Brulee (see recipe page 140)
Snacks: Slice fruit loaf
Fresh fruit

Swap refined carbs – such as white pasta or white rice – for soba noodles or wholewheat grains and you'll feel fuller for longer.

Day 9

Breakfast: Banana and Blueberry Smoothie (see recipe page 142) served with heaped teaspoonful wheatgerm
Lunch: Baked Sweet Potato with Feta, Chilli, Coriander and Toasted Pumpkin Seeds (see recipe page 133)
Dinner: Sea Bass with Chinese Greens and Oyster Sauce (see recipe page 122) served on a bed of brown rice
Mixed fruit salad
Snacks: Rice cakes with cottage cheese
Orange or nectarines

Avoid drinking tea with your meals – it can reduce the absorption of iron in the body.

Day 10

Breakfast: Fruit Pancakes (see recipe page 139)
Cup of herbal or green tea
Lunch: Turkey on a wholewheat roll and mixed salad drizzled with flaxseed oil
Fresh fruit
Dinner: Mackerel with Mustard and Lemon (see recipe page 123) served with new potatoes or Trout with Brown Rice, Spinach, Lime and Ginger Pilaf (see recipe page 121)
Snacks: Small bag apricots
Slice of pumpernickel bread with cottage cheese and pineapple

Swap fatty processed dressings for flaxseed oil – it's rich in heart-friendly fats.

Team carbohydrates with a protein source; together they'll give you a longer-lasting source of energy.

Replace fatty meats with beans in your stews and you'll get less saturated fat and more fibre in your diet.

Whipping up a quick stir fry? Pop in some broccoli and mushrooms – their disease-fighting nutrients work better when you combine them.

Want to sweeten that fruit salad? Use energy-boosting honey instead of sugar which will give you a high followed sharply by an energy-slump!

Day 11

Breakfast: Dried Fruit Compote (see recipe page 112) served with pot of natural yoghurt
Cup of herbal tea
Lunch: Spiced Chickpea Salad (see recipe page 136)
Dinner: Baked potato with roast or grilled chicken served with Rocket, Spinach and Avocado Salad (see recipe page 137)
Snacks: Matchbox-piece edam or feta cheese
Handful grapes or berries

Day 12

Breakfast: Exotic Fruit Salad with Ginger and Citrus (see recipe page 111)
Lunch: Veggie Bean Stew (see recipe page 132)
Dinner: Homemade ratatouille served with brown Basmati rice and crumbled feta
Natural fromage frais and sprinkling dried fruit
Snacks: Small pot rice pudding
Savoury Hummus with Pine Nuts (see recipe page 113)

Day 13

Breakfast: Warm Berry Compote with Vanilla and Honeyed Yoghurt (see recipe page 112)
Lunch: Tofu burger served with large mixed green salad
Apple
Dinner: Wild Rice and Borlotti Beans with Prunes and Sage (see recipe page 130)
Snacks: Rice cakes with cottage cheese
Fresh pineapple slices

Day 14

Breakfast: Bowl of oat-based cereal topped with crushed flaxseeds
Glass fresh orange juice
Lunch: Pasta with Hazelnut and Basil Pesto (see recipe page 134)
Dinner: Baked cod served with boiled new potatoes and mixed leafy green salad drizzled with olive oil
Baked apple with spoonful of honey and dollop of natural fromage frais
Snacks: Spiced Roasted Nuts (see recipe page 115)
Piece of fresh fruit

Week 3

Day 15

Breakfast: Low-fat natural yoghurt with granola and grated apple
Cup of green tea
Lunch: Tuna Nicoise Salad (see recipe page 138)
Dinner: Grilled steak with broccoli, baked sweet potato
Fruit jelly and fresh strawberries
Snacks: Slice toast with peanut butter
Sliced papaya

Green tea is a good alternative to coffee – it's thought to help increase your metabolic rate.

Day 16

Breakfast: Oat Banana Pecan Muffins
Glass fresh orange juice
Lunch: Pasta with Broccoli, Lemon, Anchovies and Chilli (see recipe page 135)
Bowl berries
Dinner: Cinnamon Chicken Breast Stuffed with Bulghur Wheat (see recipe page 129)
Melon and Peach Smoothie (see recipe on page 142)
Snacks: Handful cashew nuts
Apple

A bowl of berries is a great way to get some brain-protecting antioxidants into your diet.

Day 17

Breakfast: Poached egg and grilled tomatoes on slice wholemeal toast
Glass orange juice
Lunch: Savoury Hummus with Pine Nuts (see recipe page 113) served with large plate of crudités
Pot fromage frais
Dinner: Baked Sweet Potato with Feta, Chilli, Coriander and Toasted Pumpkin Seeds (see recipe page 133)
Snacks: Slices fresh mango
Glass skimmed milk

Want to make a simple salad more filling and nutritious? Sprinkle some nuts or seeds over the top and you'll get some brain-boosting omega-3 fatty acids into the bargain.

Want to cut down on salt? Use herbs and spices, or lemon juice instead – it adds flavour without the damage.

Day 18

Breakfast: Seeded Granola with Maple Syrup, Coconut and Dried Fruit (see recipe page 110)

Lunch: Puy Lentil Soup with Pumpkin and Fennel (see recipe page 117)

Dinner: Stir-fried vegetables with cashews or slices grilled chicken served on a bed of brown rice

Strawberries in Red Wine (see recipe page 141)

Snacks: Fruit Pancake (see recipe page 139)

Crudités with spoonful hummus

Sweet tooth? A slice of fruit loaf is a better choice than cake – it's full of iron-rich dried fruit, good for energy.

Day 19

Breakfast: Dried Fruit Compote (see recipe page 112) served with granola

Lunch: Large mixed salad drizzled with flaxseed oil, served with tinned tuna and a wholemeal pitta

Fruit yoghurt

Dinner: Roasted Soy Chicken with Sesame Seeds (see recipe page 127) served on a plate of soba noodles

Snacks: Slice fruit loaf

Bowl fresh berries

Apricots are a great on-the-go snack – rich in energy-boosting iron.

Day 20

Breakfast: Porridge served with diced dried apricots and raisins

Lunch: Pasta with Hazelnut and Basil Pesto (see recipe page 134)

Dinner: Wild Rice and Borlotti Beans with Prunes and Sage (see recipe page 130)

Fruit Brulee (recipe recipe page 140)

Snacks: Glass milk

Rice cakes with cottage cheese

Are you drinking enough water? Dehydration is linked with poor concentration. Add lemon or lime to liven up those 6–8 glasses a day.

Day 21

Breakfast: Exotic Fruit Salad with Ginger and Citrus (see recipe page 111)

Cup of herbal or green tea

Lunch: Large mozzarella, avocado and tomato salad served with slice of seedy bread

Dinner: Roasted vegetables over a bed of couscous sprinkled with feta cheese

Dried Fruit Compote (see recipe page 112)

Snacks: Handful sunflower seeds

Banana and Blueberry Smoothie (see recipe page 142)

Week 4

Day 22

Breakfast: Porridge sprinkled with handful of raisins

Cup of green tea

Lunch: Stir-fried vegetables served with toasted cashews

Fruit yoghurt

Dinner: Seared Tuna with Basil, Tomato and Anchovy salsa served with new potatoes (see recipe page 126)

Snacks: Slice pumpernickel bread with hummus

Piece fruit

Day 23

Breakfast: 2 pieces fruit, natural bio yoghurt, handful nuts

Cup of green tea

Lunch: Quinoa and Basmati Pilaff with Dill and Roasted Tomatoes (see recipe page 131)

Dinner: Veggie Bean Stew served on a bed of brown rice (see recipe page 132)

Snacks: Mixed fruit salad with small natural yoghurt

Slice fruit loaf

Day 24

Breakfast: Poached egg and grilled tomato on slice pumpernickel toast

Glass fruit juice

Piece fresh fruit

Lunch: Sweet Pea and Avocado Soup (see recipe page 116) served with mixed green salad drizzled with flaxseed oil

Dinner: Spiced Chickpea Salad (see recipe page 136) with a large baked sweet potato as a side serving

Strawberries in Red Wine (see recipe page 141)

Snacks: Handful of dried fruits and nuts

Sliced pineapple

Have you started your brain-boosting exercise regime? Make sure you're getting enough protein in your diet to help repair and heal tired muscles. Lean chicken, fish and hummus are good sources.

Having some fish? Try some yoghurt for pudding. It's thought that essential fatty acids boost absorption of calcium.

Fish for supper? Serve it with broccoli or spinach, good sources of folate; experts say folate is best absorbed with food containing vitamin B12 – such as fish.

Today's breakfast combo of seeds and vitamin C rich blueberries boosts the body's absorption of the vitamin E from the seeds.

Day 25

Breakfast: Muesli cereal sprinkled with crushed flaxseeds and blueberries
Small glass fruit juice
Lunch: Open sandwich on wholemeal, rye or pumpernickel bread with hummus and large mixed salad
2 pieces fresh fruit
Dinner: Mediterranean Tuna with Baked Sweet Potato (see recipe page 125) or Teriyaki Salmon (see recipe page 118)
Snacks: Rice pudding
Banana

Eating betacarotene rich foods (such as butternut squash) with a bit of healthy fat helps your body absorb the nutrient.

Day 26

Breakfast: Warm Berry Compote with Vanilla and Honeyed Yoghurt (see recipe page 125)
Lunch: Savoury Hummus with Pine Nuts (see recipe page 113) and crudités
Fruit jelly
Dinner: Cumin Spiced Chicken with Roasted Butternut Squash and Broccoli (see recipe page 128) served on a bed of brown rice
Snacks: Bowl raspberries
Rice cakes and cottage cheese

Pumpkin seeds are a good source of zinc. Making sure you have good intakes of protein in your diet improves absorption of this mineral.

Day 27

Breakfast: Melon and Peach Smoothie (see recipe page 142)
Boiled egg on pumpernickel toast
Lunch: Pasta with Hazelnut and Basil Pesto (see recipe page 134)
Bowl strawberries and natural yoghurt
Dinner: Baked Sweet Potato with Feta, Chilli, Coriander and Toasted Pumpkin Seeds (see recipe page 133)
Snacks: Half an avocado filled with pine nuts drizzled with olive oil
Piece of fruit

Swap fizzy cola for fresh juices, herbal teas or water while on the brain boosting eating plan. Large amounts of cola reduce your body's levels of calcium, which you need for strong bones and healthy nerve function.

Day 28

Breakfast: Melon and Peach Smoothie (see recipe page 142)
Lunch: Puy Lentil Soup with Pumpkin and Fennel (see recipe page 117)
Dinner: Haddock Wrapped in Bacon with Anchovy, Rosemary and Lemon (see recipe page 120) served with new potatoes
Fruit Brulee (see recipe page 140)
Snacks: Matchbox piece of cheddar or feta
Bowl fresh berries

The recipes
Breakfasts

Breakfast can increase your energy levels, improve your concentration and boost your mood, all of which means you're more likely to be firing on all cylinders.

Oat Banana Pecan Muffins

Makes 10–12 muffins

180g (6 1/2oz) wholemeal flour
1 tbsp baking powder
1/4 tsp salt
85g (3 1/2oz) chilled butter, cut into cubes
140g (5oz) light muscovado sugar
40g (1 1/2oz) rolled oats
50g (1 3/4oz) pecans, roughly chopped
1 large banana, finely diced
1 large egg, lightly beaten
170ml (6 fl oz) milk
1 tsp vanilla extract

1. Pre heat oven to 200°C, fan 190°C, gas 6. Grease a 12-hole muffin tin (or use muffin cases and place into the holes in the tin).
2. In a large bowl, mix together the flour, baking powder and salt. Using the tips of your fingers rub the butter into the flour until it resembles fine breadcrumbs. Stir in the sugar, oats, pecans and banana.
3. In a separate bowl mix together the egg, milk and vanilla. Make a well in the centre of the flour and pour in the liquid ingredients. Mix with a fork until just combined, being careful not to over mix.
4. Fill the muffin cups (or cases) about 3/4 full and bake for 18–20 minutes until lightly golden or a skewer inserted comes out with moist crumbs attached. Cool for 10 mins. Best eaten on the day but will keep in an airtight container for 24 hours.

Nutrition tip:

Pecans, like other nuts, are rich in omega-3 fatty acids which are important for brain function. They're also rich in zinc, which is good for the immune system to help keep body and mind healthy.

Seeded Granola with Maple Syrup, Coconut and Dried Fruit

Makes 16 servings

2 tbsp linseed oil or sunflower oil
150ml (5 1/2 fl oz) maple syrup
300g (10oz) rolled oats
100g (4oz) mixed seeds, e.g. linseeds, sunflower seeds, pumpkin seeds
4 tbsp sesame seeds
100g (4oz) flaked almonds
100g (4oz) dried fruit such as mixed berries, apricots, prunes, figs, roughly chopped
50g (2oz) desiccated coconut

To serve: milk or yoghurt

1. Heat oven to 150°C, fan 140°C, gas 2. Mix together the oil and maple syrup in a large bowl. Add all the remaining ingredients except the dried fruit and coconut, and mix well.
2. Pour the granola on to TWO baking sheets and spread evenly. Bake for 15 minutes, and then mix in the coconut and fruit. Bake for 10 minutes more, remove and scrape on to a flat tray to cool. Serve with cold milk or yoghurt. Store in an airtight container.

Nutrition tip

Oats are among the best foods for providing energy. They're rich in iron, and contain B vitamins which help lift your mood.

Exotic Fruit Salad with Ginger and Citrus

Makes 4 servings

1 orange
1 pink or red grapefruit
1 small mango
1 banana, sliced
2 kiwi, peeled and sliced
Seeds from 1 pomegranate (optional)
Thumbnail fresh ginger, peeled and finely chopped or grated
Juice of 2 limes
1/2 tbsp sugar

1. To segment the orange, cut the skin off with a serrated knife, then, holding the fruit over a bowl, cut between the membrane to remove the segments. Squeeze out the juice and repeat with the grapefruit.
2. For the mango, slice the 2 'lobes' either side of the skin. Take a sharp knife and criss-cross the skin down to the flesh. Hold the mango over the bowl and slip a tablespoon behind and as close to the skin and all the cubes of mango will fall out. Stir in the banana, kiwi and pomegranate.
3. Mix together the ginger and lime and add a little sugar to taste. Add to the fruit, let marinade for 30 minutes or so, check the sweetness, adding a little more sugar if need be, and serve.

Nutrition tip:

Citrus fruits are rich in vitamin C, a disease-fighting antioxidant, which also aids the absorption of iron. It is also involved in healthy neurological function.

Warm Berry Compote with Vanilla and Honeyed Yoghurt

Makes 4 servings

500g (18oz) mixed berries, fresh or frozen
Soft brown sugar (optional)
A little orange zest

To serve: Greek yoghurt, Manuka honey

1. Place the berries in a small pan; add a squeeze of orange and a little sugar to taste (this will depend on the sweetness of the fruit). Simmer for 2 minutes.
2. Cool slightly and serve with some Greek yoghurt and a drizzle of honey.

Dried Fruit Compote

Makes 6–8 servings

400g (16oz) dried fruit, such as: 100g (4oz) apricots, 100g (4oz) prunes, 100g (4oz) figs, 100g (4oz) cranberries or raisins
200ml (7 fl oz) apple juice
A cinnamon stick
A dollop of honey

To serve: yoghurt and/or cereal or granola

1. Place the fruit in a small pan and just cover with boiling water. Add the apple juice, cinnamon stick and a tablespoon of honey, bring to the boil and simmer for 10 minutes or so until the fruit is softened, and the juice is a little syrupy.
2. Serve warm with yoghurt or chilled for breakfast with whole-wheat cereal, granola or porridge. Will keep in the fridge for up to a week.

Snacks

Snacks are an important part of any healthy eating plan. That's because eating small regular meals helps avoid the blood sugar dips that cause lethargy, tiredness and poor concentration. If you provide your body with regular supplies of nutrients, you'll feel sharper and brighter.

Savoury Hummus with Pine Nuts

Makes 2–4 servings

410g tin chickpeas
1 tbsp tahini
2 cloves garlic, crushed
Juice 1 lemon
4 tbsp extra virgin olive oil
1 tsp marmite
2 tbsp pine nuts, toasted

To serve: cucumber, carrot, celery and pepper, cut into sticks; warm flat breads

1. Place the chickpeas, tahini paste, garlic, lemon juice, olive oil, 1 tbsp boiling water and Marmite in a food processor and whiz until very smooth. Season well.
2. Top with the nuts, and serve with the vegetable sticks and flat bread.

Nutrition tip:

Chickpeas are a good source of slow-releasing carbohydrates which provide body and mind with a good source of energy. They also provide calcium and iron which help prevent anaemia, and potassium, a mineral vital for healthy nerve impulses.

Sesame Yoghurt Dip

Makes 4 servings

55g (2oz) sesame seeds
150g (5 1/2oz) Greek yoghurt
125g (4 1/2oz) mayonnaise
3 tbsp dark soy sauce

To serve: pitta bread, crudités

1. In a dry frying pan over a moderate heat, toast the sesame seeds, stirring until they are golden. Transfer to a bowl and allow to cool completely.
2. Combine the yoghurt, mayonnaise and soy sauce and mix thoroughly. Lastly add the sesame seeds.
3. Serve with crunchy vegetables or as a topping for baked sweet potatoes with salad or roasted sweet potato wedges. This is best eaten soon after making, as the sesame seeds tend to go soggy.

Nutrition tip:

Sesame seeds are a good vegetable source of iron, which is needed for healthy brain tissue. They're also a good source of essential fatty acids, important for brain development.

Spiced Roasted Nuts

Makes 4 servings

5 tbsp dark soy sauce
A good squeeze of lemon juice
1/2 tsp sugar
8 drops of Tabasco
1 tbsp paprika
200g (7oz) mixed nuts such as walnuts, Brazils, almonds, macadamias
55g (2oz) sunflower seeds
55g (2oz) pumpkin seeds
25g (1oz) sesame seeds

1. Heat the oven to 190°C, fan 170°C, gas 5. In a bowl whisk together the soy, lemon juice, sugar, Tabasco and paprika. Stir in the nuts and seeds and coat evenly. Spread in a single layer on a baking tray and roast, stirring every 2 minutes, until golden, about 10 minutes. Do not leave unattended as they catch easily.
2. Cool completely, transfer to a bowl and enjoy as a snack or sprinkle on to a salad. Store in an airtight container.

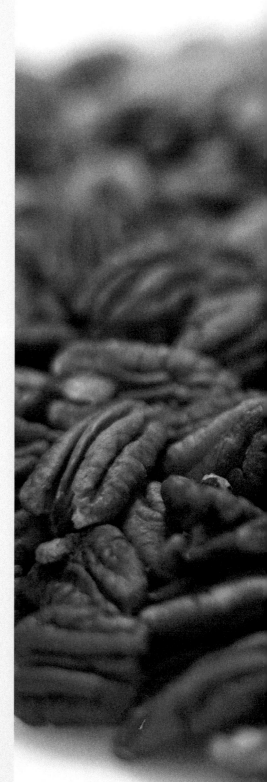

Nutrition tip:

Walnuts are a good source of omega-3 fatty acids, important for brain function, and provide B vitamins, which are needed for energy. They're also rich in vitamin E, which helps protect your nerves from the ageing process.

Soups

Soup makes a nutritious lunch, starter or snack. Soup can also be a good way to incorporate a wide range of vegetables in your diet, and may keep you fuller for longer – and lose pounds as a result. If your mind is preoccupied as a result of cravings, try incorporating more nutritious soups into your diet. Researchers at the University of Pennsylvania found that when people start a meal with soup as a first course, they tend to end up consuming fewer calories.

Sweet Pea and Avocado Soup

Makes 4 servings

1 large ripe avocado, pitted, peeled and cubed
150g (5 1/2oz) frozen peas, thawed
560ml (1 pt) chicken or vegetable stock
3 spring onions, chopped
3 tbsp lemon or limejuice
2 tbsp Greek yoghurt or sour cream
Handful cherry tomatoes, chopped
Small handful coriander roughly chopped
1 tbsp extra virgin olive oil or flaxseed oil
Squeeze of lemon juice

1. In a liquidiser or food processor combine the peas and avocado until very smooth.
2. Add the stock, lemon juice, yoghurt or sour cream and blend again. Season well.
3. Mix together the tomatoes, oil and lemon. Serve the soup, with a spoonful of salsa on top.

Nutrition tip:

Avocados are rich in mono-unsaturated fat which has been found to help preserve our mental abilities as we age. It's also rich in disease-fighting antioxidant vitamin E.

Eat Yourself Clever Carol Vorderman

Puy Lentil Soup with Pumpkin and Fennel

Makes 4 servings

4 tbsp olive oil
1 onion, peeled and finely chopped
1 fennel bulb, tough outer layer removed, halved and finely chopped
180g (6 1/2oz) Puy lentils
1 tsp fennel seeds
2 litres (3 1/2 pts) chicken or vegetable stock
240g (8oz) or 1/2 medium butternut squash, peeled and cut into small cubes
Handful flat leaf parsley, roughly chopped

1. Heat the oil and sauté the onion and fennel until softened, about 10 minutes. Add the lentils and fennel seeds, pour over the stock, bring to the boil and simmer for 30 minutes.
2. Add the squash and half the parsley and simmer gently for another 20 minutes until all the vegetables and lentils are thoroughly cooked.
3. To season: add a squeeze of lemon juice and stir in the rest of the parsley. Serve with a drizzle of extra virgin oil, or puree if you prefer a smoother texture.

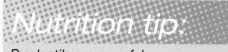

Nutrition tip:

Puy lentils are a useful source of protein and iron which provides energy for your body and mind.

Main courses
Fish dishes

Fish is a key ingredient in any healthy eating plan. Oily fish is rich in brain-boosting omega-3 fatty acids, and white fish is a lean source of protein which contains important nutrients.

Teriyaki Salmon

Makes 4 servings

6 tbsp teriyaki marinade
2 tsp sesame, flaxseed or sunflower oil
Thumbnail fresh ginger, peeled and grated
Zest of 2 limes
4 salmon steaks, approx 150g (5 1/2oz)

To serve: soba noodles, pickled ginger and wasabi

1. Combine the teriyaki, ginger, oil and lime zest. Pour over the salmon and marinade for at least 30 minutes at room temperature or up to 6 hours in the fridge.
2. Preheat the grill to high, place the salmon on a foil-lined grill pan and cook for 5–6 minutes until almost cooked through.
3. Leave to rest for 5 minutes whereby the fish will continue to cook slightly and have a delicious velvety texture. (You can always cook a little more if you find it too rare.) Serve with soba noodles, pickled ginger and wasabi. This marinade also works well with tuna.

Nutrition tip:

Salmon is very rich in omega-3 fatty acids which have been found to play an important role in memory and brain function.

Filo Parcels with Salmon and Feta

Makes 4 servings

2 x 220g (8oz) packs washed spinach leaves
A little freshly grated nutmeg
Finely grated zest and juice of 1 lemon
8 sheets filo pastry
4 salmon fillets, approx 150g (5 1/2oz) each
150g (5 1/2oz) feta cheese, crumbled
55g (2oz) butter, melted

To serve: dressed leaf salad

1. Heat the oven to 220°C, fan 210°C, gas 7. Cook the spinach in a large pan with a couple of tablespoons of water until just wilted. Drain well in a colander and squeeze out the excess moisture. Season with salt, pepper, nutmeg and the lemon zest and juice.
2. Take 2 sheets of filo (keep the rest under a damp tea towel to stop it drying out). Brush one with butter and pop the other on top. Place the salmon on the bottom half, top with 1/4 of the spinach, press down and top with the feta. Brush the edges of the filo with butter, flip the sides and bottom of the pastry over the salmon and roll up to make a parcel.
3. Repeat with the others and put on to a baking tray. Brush each parcel with the butter and bake for 15 minutes until crisp and golden.
4. Serve immediately so that the salmon does not overcook.

Nutrition tip:

Spinach is a great vegetable source of iron, important for keeping anaemia and associated mental tiredness at bay. It's also rich in disease-fighting antioxidants to keep your cells healthy.

Haddock Wrapped in Bacon with Anchovy, Rosemary and Lemon

Makes 4 servings

4 anchovy fillets
1 tbsp fresh rosemary, finely chopped
Finely grated zest and juice of 1 lemon
2 tbsp extra virgin olive oil
4 haddock fillets, approx 150g (5 1/2oz) each
8 slices thinly sliced lean bacon or Parma ham

To serve: broccoli, green beans or Savoy cabbage

1. Preheat the oven to 200°C, fan 190°C, gas 6. Mix together the anchovy, rosemary, lemon zest, juice and olive oil. Season the fish fillets and wrap 2 pieces of the bacon around each fillet.
2. Place on a tray and roast in the oven for 5 minutes, then remove and drizzle over some of the anchovy dressing. Return to the oven for another 5 minutes. The fish should be opaque when pierced with a knife and the bacon slightly crisped. Serve with the vegetables of your choice.

Nutrition tip:

White fish such as haddock is a good lean source of protein, and rich in B vitamins important for healthy nerve and brain cell function.

Eat Yourself Clever Carol Vorderman

Trout with Brown Rice, Spinach, Lime and Ginger Pilaf

Makes 4 servings

4 x skinless trout or salmon fillets, approx 150g (5 1/2oz) each
1/4 tsp mild chilli powder
2 tbsp flaxseed or olive oil
1 red onion, sliced
4 garlic cloves, finely chopped
200g (7oz) brown Basmati rice
500ml (18 fl oz) light chicken stock
Thumbnail fresh ginger, peeled and grated
Zest of 2 limes
100g (1/2 bag) baby spinach
Small handful fresh coriander

1. Preheat the grill. Place the fish on some foil, sprinkle over the chilli powder, half the lime zest and all the juice and season.
2. Heat a large sauté pan with a lid and sauté the onion until softened, add the garlic and rice, pour over the hot stock, cover and simmer very gently until the rice is cooked and the stock absorbed. Add a little more water if the rice is not quite cooked.
3. Stir in the freshly grated ginger and the remaining lime zest. Add the spinach, cover and cook for a further 3–4 minutes, then stir through to wilt. Season to taste. Serve with the grilled fish and scatter over the coriander. Also good with grilled chicken.

Nutrition tip:

Brown Basmati rice is a good source of complex carbohydrates which help provide your body and mind with a longer-lasting supply of energy.

Sea Bass with Chinese Greens and Oyster Sauce

Makes 4 servings

4 sea bass fillets, approx 150g (5 1/2oz) each
2 tsp sesame oil
4 handfuls chopped greens, such as spinach, pak choy, broccoli and rocket
2 tsp flaxseed or sunflower oil
1 thumbnail ginger, grated
2 mild red chillies, de-seeded and finely chopped
2 cloves garlic, finely chopped
4 tbsp oyster sauce
4 tbsp teriyaki sauce

1. Season the fish and place the fish on a foil-lined grill pan. Drizzle with a tsp of the sesame oil and cook under a hot grill for 4–5 minutes until the flesh is just opaque. Wrap the foil around the fish, and allow to rest; it will carry on cooking slightly.
2. Steam or blanch the greens for 2–3 minutes, until just cooked but still retaining some crunch. Meanwhile heat the oils, add the ginger, chillies and garlic and cook for 2 minutes. Stir in the oyster sauce and teriyaki and heat through. Add the greens, mix well and serve with the fish.

Nutrition tip:

Leafy green veg are full of vitamin C, important for healthy cells. They're also a great source of folic acid, a lack of which has been linked to depression – which also affects your mental energy.

Eat Yourself Clever Carol Vorderman

Mackerel with Mustard and Lemon

Makes 4 servings

4 fresh mackerel, each weighing about 250g (9oz), cleaned and gutted
4 tbsp mild wholegrain mustard
25g (1oz) unsalted butter
3 tbsp single cream
Olive oil

To serve: lemon wedges, watercress salad dressed with lemon and olive oil

1. Make cuts at diagonals along each side of the fish. Rub 2 tbsp of the mustard over the skin of the fish and into the slashes.
2. To make the sauce melt the butter in a small pan and cook the mustard for a couple of minutes. Add the cream, stir and season to taste; the sauce should be thick. Set to one side and keep warm.
3. Lightly oil the fish and griddle or grill for about 6 minutes per side until lightly charred and the flesh is cooked through to the bone (to check, the flesh should feel firm to the touch). Serve the fish with a spoonful of the sauce and the watercress salad.

Nutrition tip:

Mackerel is an oily fish, rich in brain-boosting omega-3 fatty acids. It also provides vitamin D, which is important for a healthy nervous system, and iron.

Grilled Sardines with Sicilian Flavours

Makes 4 servings

8 large or 12 medium very fresh sardines, cleaned and gutted
55g (2oz) pine nuts
Handful parsley, roughly chopped
1 tbsp currants or raisins
Zest of 1 small orange
Zest of 1 lemon
3 tbsp freshly made breadcrumbs
2 tbsp olive oil

To serve: lemon wedges, dressed mixed salad, new potatoes

1. Pre heat the oven to 200°C, fan 190°C, gas 6. Place the sardines in a roasting tray or shallow oven dish, laying them out in a single layer. Mix together the nuts, parsley, currants, zest and breadcrumbs and sprinkle around and on top of the fish.
2. Drizzle over the olive oil and cook in the oven for 8–10 minutes, depending on the size of the fish, until cooked through (i.e. the flesh is opaque when pierced with a knife.) Serve with lemon wedges, a simple salad and potatoes.

Nutrition tip:

Sardines provide useful amounts of the nutrient choline, which is linked to memory and mental function. Choline helps your brain's neurotransmitters work efficiently.

Mediterranean Tuna with Baked Sweet Potato

Makes 4 servings

Finely grated zest of 1 lemon
2 cloves garlic, crushed
2 tsp fennel seeds
2 tbsp olive oil
4 tuna steaks, approx 150g (5 1/2oz) each
4 medium sweet potatoes

To serve: broccoli or rocket salad

1. Preheat the to oven 180°C, fan 170°C, gas 4. Mix together the lemon zest, garlic, fennel seeds and olive oil. Smear all over the tuna and leave to marinade for about 30 minutes. Bake the sweet potatoes for 45 minutes, until soft in the middle when pierced with a knife.
2. Heat a non-stick pan or griddle pan until searing hot and cook the tuna for just 2 minutes on the first side and 1 minute on the second side or until cooked to your liking. Serve with the sweet potatoes and steamed broccoli or rocket salad.

Nutrition tip:

Sweet potatoes are a rich source of the antioxidant vitamins C and E and betacarotene, which help protect your cells from disease and decline. They're also a good source of slow-releasing carbohydrates.

Seared Tuna with Basil, Tomato and Anchovy Salsa

Makes 4 servings

4 tuna steaks, approx 150g (5 1/2oz) each
4 anchovy fillets in oil, drained and finely chopped
200g (7oz) punnet cherry tomatoes, chopped
1 clove garlic, finely chopped
1 tbsp capers
Small handful basil, finely chopped
Extra virgin olive oil

To serve: new potatoes

1. Mix together the anchovy, tomatoes, garlic, capers and basil. Add enough oil to loosen and season to taste.
2. Heat a griddle pan until searing hot. Lightly oil the tuna and cook for 2 minutes on the first side, without moving, so that the fish doesn't stick. Cook for a further 1–2 minutes on the second side for medium-rare. Serve with the salsa spooned over with some new potatoes.

Nutrition tip:

Tomatoes are full of the antioxidant lycopene which is known for its anti-ageing properties.

Chicken dishes
Roasted Soy Chicken with Sesame Seeds

Makes 4 servings

2 thumbnails fresh ginger, peeled and grated
2 tbsp caster sugar
125ml (4 1/2 fl oz) oyster sauce
125ml (4 1/2 fl oz) dry sherry
1 tsp sesame oil
4 x chicken breasts
4 spring onions, sliced

To serve: toasted sesame seeds, rice and/or Mange tout or any dark green leafy vegetables

1. Place the ginger, sugar, oyster sauce, sherry and sesame oil in a bowl and combine. Add the chicken and marinade for at least 30 minutes at room temperature and up to 12 hours in the fridge. (But always bring the chicken to room temperature for about 30 minutes before cooking.)
2. Pre heat the oven to 220°C, fan 200°C, gas 7. Place chicken on a roasting tray in the oven for 10–12 minutes until just cooked through. Serve sprinkled with sesame seeds, spring onions and the vegetables of your choice.

Nutrition tip:

Lean chicken is a nutritious, low-fat source of protein. It contains iron and magnesium (which is linked to mood) and is rich in the amino acid tyrosine which produces the brain chemicals dopamine and noradrenaline, which can boost concentration and mental alertness.

Cumin Spiced Chicken with Roasted Butternut Squash and Broccoli

Makes 4 servings

8 chicken thighs
2 tsp cumin seeds
2 tsp coriander seeds, crushed
Olive oil
1 butternut squash, cut into chunks
2 heads broccoli, cut into florets, stalks peeled and sliced
Small handful coriander

To serve: Greek yoghurt tzatziki

1. Preheat the oven to 200°C, fan 190°C, gas 6. Spread the squash in a roasting tin in a single layer and place the thighs on top. Sprinkle over the spices and drizzle over the olive oil. Try to distribute everything evenly.
2. Pop into the oven to roast for about 20 minutes. Add the broccoli and garlic to the tray, stir everything a little bit to make sure it all cooks evenly, then return it to the oven for a further 15 minutes or so until the chicken is cooked and the vegetables are tender and beginning to char around the edges.
3. Serve scattered with coriander and a spoonful of tzatziki.

Nutrition tip:

Butternut squash is rich in disease-fighting carotenes which help fight the free radicals that cause our body – including the brain – to age.

Cinnamon Chicken Breasts Stuffed with Bulghur Wheat

Makes 4 servings

4 boneless chicken breasts, skin on, approx 180g (6 1/2oz) each
1 large onion, thinly sliced
2 cloves garlic, chopped
Thumbnail ginger, peeled and chopped
3 tbsp olive oil
1 tsp cinnamon
1 tsp garam masala
20g pack coriander
50g (2oz) toasted almonds
30g (1oz) sultanas
100g (4oz) bulghur wheat

To serve: green beans, cabbage or broccoli

1. Heat oven to 200°C, fan 170°C, gas 6. Heat 2 tbsp of the oil, fry onion, ginger and garlic for 6–8 minutes until soft, add the spices and sauté 2 minutes more.
2. Boil the bulghur wheat and sultanas for 5 minutes until soft and add to the onion mix. Mix in the coriander and almonds and season.
3. Cut chicken breasts to open like a book and divide stuffing between them (there may be some left over to serve alongside). Fold the chicken back over and place in a small baking dish. Drizzle over the rest of the oil and bake for 20 minutes until the chicken is cooked through. Serve with vegetables of your choice.

Nutrition tip:

Bulghur wheat is an excellent source of complex carbohydrate which keeps you fuller for longer, and less prone to drops in sugar levels which cause fatigue. Wholegrains such as bulghur wheat also contain B vitamins, important for cognitive skills and memory.

Vegetarian dishes
Wild Rice and Borlotti Beans with Prunes and Sage

Makes 4 servings

200g (7 1/2oz) wild rice
1 x 410g can borlotti beans, drained and rinsed
4 tbsp extra virgin olive oil
1 large red onion, finely chopped
4 cloves garlic, finely chopped
2 sprigs sage
55g (2oz) stoned prunes
150g (6 1/2oz) pecan nuts, lightly toasted

To serve: spinach or rocket salad dressed with lemon and olive oil

1. Cook the wild rice in plenty of well-salted water until soft but not mushy, about 40 minutes.
2. Heat the oil and sauté the onion for a few minutes then add the garlic and sage and cook for 3–4 minutes more.
3. Add the drained beans and prunes and cooked rice and stir together well. Cook for 5 minutes for all the flavours to mingle. Lastly stir through the pecans and serve with the salad. Also great with roast chicken.

Nutrition tip:

Prunes are one of the richest sources of antioxidants, and outperform other fruits for their disease-fighting properties. They also provide iron and fibre, and potassium.

Quinoa and Basmati Pilaff with Dill and Roasted Tomatoes

Makes 4 servings

250g (9oz) cherry tomatoes, halved
5 tbsp olive oil
1 onion, thinly sliced
3 sticks celery, sliced
2 garlic cloves, finely chopped
1/2 tsp cumin seeds, crushed
140g (5oz) quinoa
100g (4oz) Basmati rice (brown or white)
500ml (18 fl oz) vegetable stock
2 x 20g packs dill

To serve: handful toasted pine nuts, thick Greek yoghurt

1. Heat oven to 180°C, fan 170°C, gas 4. Place tomatoes on a baking sheet and drizzle with 2 tbsp of the olive oil and season. Roast for 15 minutes and set aside.
2. Heat the rest of the olive oil in a saucepan. Sauté the onion, celery, garlic and cumin for a few minutes until softened. Add the quinoa and dry fry the seeds with the onion mix to give them a toasty flavour.
3. Add the rice and stock, stir everything together well, cover and simmer slowly for about 25 minutes until all the liquid is absorbed and the rice cooked. Add a dash more water if need be.
4. Stir through the dill and serve topped with the nuts and a spoonful of yoghurt. Great with grilled fish and chicken too.

Nutrition tip:

Quinoa provides complex carbohydrates and some protein, so it's a good filling food. It also contains minerals such as iron.

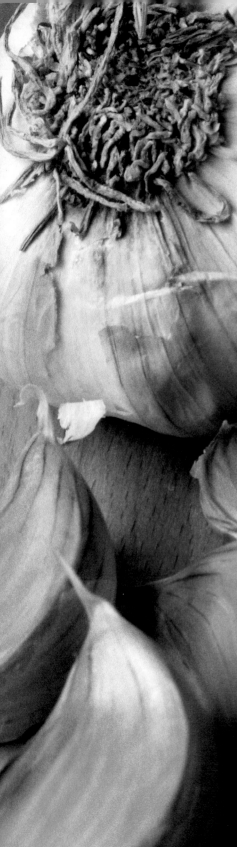

Veggie Bean Stew

Makes 4 servings

1 large onion, roughly chopped
3 garlic cloves, finely chopped
100ml (3 1/2fl oz) fino/dry sherry
2 cans beans such as flageolet, canellini, butter beans or borlotti, drained and rinsed
4 vine tomatoes, roughly chopped
2 bay leaves
600ml (1 pint) vegetarian stock
Handful of chopped parsley

To serve: crusty bread

1. Heat the oil and sauté the onion for 2–3 minutes until softened, add the garlic and cook until the onion is golden.
2. Add the sherry and let bubble away. Add the beans, chopped vine tomatoes and stock and simmer for 10–15 minutes until reduced and tasty. Season and serve sprinkled with the parsley and lots of crusty bread to mop up the juices

Nutrition tip:

Beans are good sources of protein, important for energy. They also contain minerals such as calcium, zinc and iron, and are high in fibre so they can help guard against digestive problems such as constipation which can make you feel sluggish.

Baked Sweet Potato with Feta, Chilli, Coriander and Toasted Pumpkin Seeds

Makes 4 servings

4 medium sweet potatoes
55g (2oz) pumpkin seeds
1/2 tbsp dark soy sauce
150g (5 1/2oz) feta cheese, crumbled
Zest of 1 lemon
Handful coriander, roughly chopped
1/2 mild red chilli, de-seeded and finely chopped
2 large handfuls baby spinach or rocket
Lemon
Extra virgin olive oil

1. Pre heat the oven to 180°C, fan 170°C, gas 4. Bake the sweet potatoes until soft in the centre when pierced with a knife, about 45 minutes.
2. Toast the pumpkin seeds in a dry pan until they begin to brown lightly and 'pop'. Off the heat sprinkle over the soy, mix well and set aside.
3. Combine the feta, lemon zest, coriander and chilli, stir through the spinach or rocket and dress with a squeeze of lemon and a glug of olive oil. Season and serve with the hot baked potatoes.

Nutrition tip:

Pumpkin seeds are a rich source of iron which can help combat anaemia. They're also rich in zinc, and contain potassium, magnesium and phosphorus.

Pasta dishes

Pasta makes a quick and easy meal. Choose wholewheat pasta and combine it with a protein source for a slower-releasing, longer-lasting supply of energy.

Pasta with Hazelnut and Basil Pesto

Makes 4 servings

350g (12oz) wholewheat tagliatelle
100g (3 1/2oz) toasted hazelnuts
2 large handfuls basil or 80g supermarket pack of basil, leaves only
55g (2oz) fresh Parmesan, grated
100ml extra virgin olive oil
Zest of 1/2 lemon
A little lemon juice

1. Cook the pasta in boiling salted water according to packet instructions (less 1–2 minutes for al dente). Drain and return to the pan.
2. Meanwhile, in a food processor or a handheld blender, whiz together the nuts, herbs, and olive oil. Whiz again briefly to incorporate the cheese. Season and add the lemon zest and a squeeze of lemon. Spoon over the pasta and mix well. Serve with extra Parmesan if you like. You can also replace the hazelnuts with walnuts or pine nuts.

Nutrition tip:

Wholewheat pasta provides a more efficient, longer-lasting source of energy than refined carbohydrates. It also provides vitamin B, important for nerve cells, and magnesium, which plays a key role in maintaining the body's energy levels.

Pasta with Broccoli, Lemon, Anchovies and Chilli

Makes 4 servings

6 anchovy fillets, chopped
4 cloves garlic, finely chopped
1 mild chilli, de-seeded and finely chopped (or pinch chilli flakes)
Finely grated zest of 1 large unwaxed lemon
350g (12oz) wholewheat pasta shapes
1 large head broccoli (about 350g/12oz), cut into florets, stalks peeled and sliced
Extra virgin olive oil

To serve: freshly grated Parmesan

1. In a medium frying pan heat a little of the anchovy oil from the tin and sauté the anchovy, garlic and chilli for 2–3 minutes. Add the lemon zest and set aside.
2. Cook the pasta according to packet instructions (less 1–2 minutes for al dente). Add the broccoli for the last 5 minutes of cooking. Check that the pasta is cooked then drain loosely. Return to the pan and add the anchovy mix. Add a good slug of olive oil and toss together well. Season and serve with a good sprinkling of Parmesan.

Nutrition tip:

Chillies contain vitamin C, potassium and some betacarotene. The hot burning flavour is caused by capsaicin, a powerful phenolic compound which has been found to have anti-cancer properties. They are also said to release feel-good endorphins which boost mood, and have been found to increase blood flow around the body.

Salads

These can make great meals as well as side dishes. Up the brain-boosting nutrient factor by adding a wide variety of vegetables, pulses, seeds and nuts.

Spiced Chickpea Salad

Makes 4 servings

2 red peppers, de-seeded and halved
2 tins chickpeas, drained and rinsed
1 small red onion, finely chopped
Handful cherry tomatoes, chopped
Handful of parsley, chopped
1 tsp each cumin and coriander seeds, crushed
Zest and juice of 1 lemon
2 cloves garlic, crushed
4 tbsp olive oil
100g (3 1/2oz) baby spinach leaves
100g (3 1/2oz) feta cheese, crumbled

1. Preheat the oven to 200°C, fan 190°C, gas 6. Roast the red peppers until charred. Cool, then peel and roughly chop. Mix together the garlic, cumin, coriander, smoked paprika, oil and lemon.
2. Heat the chickpeas briefly and add the spice marinade, peppers, cherry tomatoes and onion. Cool then add the parsley and stir through the spinach. Season and serve topped with the feta cheese.

Nutrition tip:

Red peppers are an excellent source of vitamin C, and are rich in the antioxidants betacarotene and beta-cryptoxanthin. The vitamin C content in red peppers is said to enhance the protective effects of its antioxidants.

Rocket, Spinach and Avocado Salad

Makes 4 servings

170g (6oz) baby spinach leaves
170g (6oz) rocket
2 avocados
2 small courgettes, thinly sliced
4 tbsp (60ml) extra virgin olive oil
2 tbsp (60ml) lemon juice
2 garlic cloves, finely chopped

1. Cut the avocados into quarters, remove the stones and peel. Combine the spinach and rocket in a large bowl, and add the avocado and courgette.
2. Shake the oil, lemon juice and garlic in a bottle or screw top glass jar; drizzle over the salad. Toss, then serve.

Nutrition tip:

Spinach and rocket are rich in folic acid which has been linked to a reduced risk of stroke and helps guard against dementia in later life. It has also been found to have positive effects on memory.

Tuna Nicoise Salad

Makes 4 servings

250g (10oz) new potatoes
4 fresh tuna steaks
3 medium free range eggs
75g (2 1/2oz) fine green beans
2 Little Gem lettuces
4 vine-ripened tomatoes
1 red onion, cut into fine rings
6 anchovies (optional)
10–12 black olives (stoned)

Dressing:
2 tbsp extra virgin olive oil
1 tbsp balsamic vinegar
1 tbsp white wine vinegar
1 tsp Dijon mustard
1 tsp caster sugar
Salt and black pepper
(Put all ingredients into a jar with a screw top and shake. Keeps in the fridge for up to 2 weeks.)

1. Cook the potatoes for about 15 minutes or until tender. Meanwhile, steam the beans over the top.
2. Grill or griddle the tuna for about 2–3 minutes each side, then, when slightly cooled, break into flakes.
3. Hard boil the eggs (for about 5–6 minutes so the yolks are still slightly soft). When cool, chop into quarters.
4. Arrange the lettuce, beans, onion, potatoes, tuna and tomatoes on a plate, and drizzle the dressing over the top. Add the eggs and anchovies, then use the olives to garnish.

Nutrition tip:

Eggs are a rich source of choline, a B vitamin which is needed for healthy brain cell membranes.

Puddings

Fruit Pancakes

Makes 12 small pancakes

70g (2 1/2oz) plain white flour
70g (2 1/2oz) wholemeal flour
2 large free range eggs
250ml (8 fl oz) milk
A splash of vegetable oil

Serve with sliced fresh fruit, compote, fruit purees or manuka honey.

1. Combine the flours in a bowl. Beat the eggs and milk together, and add to the flour, gradually. Alternatively, blend all of the ingredients in a liquidiser or blender until smooth.
2. Heat a pan and add a few drops of oil. Coat the bottom of the pan with batter and cook for about 1–2 minutes. The bottom of the pancake should be golden brown. Flop the pancake and cook for a further 30–60 seconds.

Nutrition tip:

Milk is a good source of protein, providing all the essential amino acids for growth and repair of the body. It contains tyrosine which the body converts into noradrenaline for mental alertness.

Fruit Brulee

Makes 4 servings

100g (4oz) fresh, ripe strawberries
80g (3oz) fresh raspberries
50g (2oz) caster sugar
Two firm but ripe peaches
2 small ripe mangoes
2 dessertspoonfuls Kirsch (optional)
350g (12oz) natural fromage frais

1. Chop the strawberries and raspberries, sprinkle them with about 10g (1/2oz) of the caster sugar.
2. Halve and stone the peaches. Remove the skin by covering them with boiling water and leaving to stand for one minute. Then skin, chop and add to the berries. Chop the mangoes and add. Sprinkle with kirsch if using.
3. Divide between four ramekin dishes or other flameproof dishes. Spoon the fromage frais over the top.
4. Sprinkle the remaining caster sugar over the top and immediately caramelise the sugar with a blowtorch. If you don't have a blowtorch, put the sugar into a small saucepan, add 2 dessertspoons cold water and stir over a moderate heat until the sugar dissolves. Bring to the boil until the syrup turns a caramel colour, then quickly drizzle the caramel over the fromage frais.
5. Chill the ramekins well until ready to serve.

Nutrition tip:

Mangoes are a good source of the antioxidant beta carotene which has been linked to a reduced risk of Alzheimer's disease.

Strawberries in Red Wine

Makes 4 servings

500g (18oz) fresh, ripe strawberries, left at room temperature
Finely zested rind of 1/2 orange
40g (1 1/2oz) fine, organic cane sugar
230 ml (8 fl oz) Cabernet Sauvignon red wine
A few strips of orange rind to decorate

1. Place the strawberries in a bowl and add the zested orange rind. Sprinkle with the sugar, add the red wine, and stir gently together. Cover and leave to soak at room temperature for 20–30 minutes, stirring occasionally.
2. Spoon the mixture into wine glasses. Decorate with strips of orange rind.

Nutrition tip:

In moderation, red wine may have positive benefits, and may help you relax, so can be a good de-stresser for the brain. Red wine is rich in cancer-fighting flavonoids, and drinking it in moderation may help protect you against Alzheimer's.

Smoothies

These make great breakfasts or snacks, and are an ideal way to increase your intake of nutrient-rich fruit and veg.

Banana and Blueberry Smoothie

Makes 4 servings

1 ripe banana
2–3 tablespoons runny honey
150g (5oz) pot natural yoghurt
250g (9oz) blueberries

1. Blend all the ingredients together. Serve immediately.

Mango, Pineapple and Ginger Smoothie

Makes 4 servings

1 ripe mango
Thumbnail fresh ginger
200g (7oz) pineapple, cut into chunks
Handful ice cubes or chopped ice

1. Peel and chop mango, grate the ginger, and combine with the other ingredients. Blend until smooth.

Melon and Peach Smoothie

Makes 4 servings

Half a cantaloupe melon
2 peaches
2 small bananas, cut into chunks
Handful ice cubes

1. Peel, seed and chop the melon and peaches, and add to other ingredients. Blend until smooth.

References

Chapter 1

Page 8: 'Believing that you can become more intelligent . . .' Blackwell L, Trzesniewski K, Dweck C: Child Development, volume 78, No.1 (2007).

Page 12: 'Deficiency in . . .' Small, MF: 'The Happy Fat', New Scientist (24 August 2002).

Chapter 2

Page 17: 'For example, one report published in 2005 . . .' Dani, Burrill, Demmig-Adams: 'The Remarkable Role of Nutrition in Learning and Behaviour', Journal of Nutrition & Food Science, volume 35, issue 4 (2005).

Page 25: 'One study . . .' Brown, M.J., Ferruzzi, M.G., Nguyen, M.L., Cooper, D.A., Eldridge, A.L., Schwartz, S.J., White, W.S. Carotenoid: 'Bioavailability is higher from salads ingested with full-fat than with fat-reduced salad dressings as measured with electrochemical detection.' The American Journal of Clinical Nutrition, 80(2): 396–40 (2004).

Page 27: 'One study from the University of the State of Mexico . . .' International Journal of Neuroscience, 1–4:113–21 (August 1999).

Page 27: 'One US study . . .' Magnesium Research, 8: 341–58 (1995).

Page 31: 'Fish oils can also be an effective mood booster.' American Journal of Psychiatry, volume 159: 477–479 (March 2002).

Page 31: 'One study . . .' Metabolism, volume 53, issue 6: 749–754 (June 2004).

Page 31: 'An Italian study of cardiac patients . . .' Circulation, 10, 1161/01 (2002).

Page 31: 'Research published in the medical journal Drug Discovery Today . . .' Drug Discovery Today, volume 9, issue 4: 165–172 (15 February 2004).

Page 31: 'Research from the University of Southern California . . .' Breast Cancer Research, 9: 201 (2006).

Page 33: 'Cutting your intake of saturated fat . . .' The Lancet, volume 362, issue 9379: 212–214 (19 July 2003).

Chapter 3

Page 41: 'Experts say that 98% of women have cravings . . .' International Journal of Eating Disorders, 29: 195–204 (2001).

Page 44: 'Research in the Journal of Reproductive Medicine . . .' Journal of Reproductive Medicine, 36(2): 131–136 (February 1991).

Page 44: 'researchers at Princeton . . .' Obesity Research, volume 10, 478.

Page 45: 'Other studies on rats . . .' Journal of Physiology – Regulatory, Integrative and Comparative Physiology

Page 49: 'One US study found that people who eat breakfast . . .' American Journal of Clinical Nutrition, volume 55, 645–651 (1992).

Page 54: 'Recent research . . .' Obesity Research, 15: 1702–1709 (2007).

Chapter 4

Page 55: 'Research from the University of Maryland . . .' Potential impact of strawberries on human health: a review of the science. Hannum, S. M., Critical Reviews in Food Science and Nutrition 2004;44(1):1-17.

Page 55: 'Researchers at Tufts University . . .' Neurobiology of Aging, volume 27, issue 2, 344–350 (February 2006).

Page 57: 'A study reported in the Annals of Neurology . . .' Nurk, E., Refsum, H., Tell, G. S., Engedal, K., Vollset, S. E., Ueland, P. M., Nygaard, H. A., Smith, A. D.: 'Plasma total homocysteine and memory in the elderly: The Hordaland Homocysteine study', Annals of Neurology 58(6): 847–857 (2005 December).

Page 59: 'A recent London study . . .' Pharmacology, Biochemistry and Behavior, volume 75, number 3: 721–729 (June 2003).

Page 60: 'research at Loughborough University . . .' British Journal of Nutrition, volume 93, issue 06: 885–893 (Jun 2005).

Page 60: 'one study of 5,000 people . . .' American Journal of Epidemiology, volume 150, No.1: 37–44.

Page 61: 'according to experts at Tufts University . . .' 'Can Foods Forestall Ageing?' Agricultural Research, volume 47, No. 2 (February 1999).

Page 61: 'One study published . . .' Kuriyama, S., Hozawa, A., Ohmori, K., Shimazu, T., Matsui, T., Ebihara, S., Awata, S., Nagatomi, R., Arai, H., Tsuji, I.: 'Green tea consumption and cognitive function: a cross-sectional study from the Tsurugaya Project', The American Journal of Clinical Nutrition, 83(2): 355–361 (February 2006).

Page 61: 'a study in the Journal of Nutrition . . .' Rogers, E.J., Milhalik, S., Ortiz, D., Shea, T.B., 'Healing and Aging', The Journal of Nutrition, 7(6): 1–6 (2003).

Page 64: 'Scientists at Harvard . . .' www.hsph.harvard.edu/nutritionsource/fruits.html

Page 65: 'According to . . .' Anita Bean: Fitness on a Plate, A&C Black (2003).

Page 66: 'One new study published in the Annals of Neurology . . .' Scarmeas, N.,
Stern, Y., Tang, M. X., Mayeux, R., Luchsinger, J. A.: 'Mediterranean diet and risk for Alzheimer's disease', Annals of Neurology, 59(6): 912–921 (June 2006).

Chapter 5

Page 69: 'Alzheimer's and weight'. Fishel, M. A., Watson, G. S. Montine, T.J., et al: 'Hyperinsulinaemia provokes synchrous increase in central inflammation and beta amyloid in normal adults', Archives of Neurology, 62 (2005).

Page 70: 'a University of Bristol study . . .' Richardson, N.J., Rogers, P.J., et al: 'Mood and performance effect of caffeine in relation to acute and chronic caffeine deprivation', Pharmacology, Biochemistry and Behavior, volume 52(2), (1995).

Page 70: 'a study published in the American Journal of Psychiatry . . .' Gilliland, K., Andress, D.: 'Ad Lib Caffeine consumption, symptoms of caffeinism and academic performance.' American Journal of Psychiatry, volume 138(4), (1981).

Page 71: 'one study showed that the additive tartrazine . . .' Ward, N. et al: Journal of Nutritional Medicine, volume 10 (1990).

Page 72: 'in one study . . .' Brown, S.A., Tapert, S.F.: 'Adolescent Trajectory of Alcohol Use', Adolescent Brain Development, Volume 1021 (June 2004).

Chapter 6

Page 78: 'Massage may help . . .' Hernandez-Reif, M., Field, T., Krasnegor, J., Theakston, T.: 'Low back pain is reduced and range of motion increased after massage therapy', International Journal of Neuroscience, 106: 131–145 (2001).

Page 81: 'One recent study from the Journal of Gerontology . . .' The Journals of Gerontology Series A: Biological Sciences and Medical Sciences, 61:1166–1170 (2006).

Page 81: 'even three 15-minute sessions . . .' Larson, E., Li Wang, E. B., Bowen, J.D., McCormick, W. C., Linda, T., Crane, P., and Kukull, W.: Annals of Internal Medicine, volume 144, issue 2: 73–81 (2006).

Page 81: 'one study from Loughborough University . . .' International Journal of Obesity, volume 24, No. 10: 1303–1309 (October 2000).

Page 82: 'One study in the journal of Behaviour Research and Therapy   ' Behaviour Research and Therapy, volume 42, issue 2: 125-136 (February 2004).

Page 85: 'research in the British Journal of Health Psychology . . .' British Journal of Health Psychology, volume 9, No. 3: 393–403 (September 2004).

Page 85: 'A study in the American Journal of Preventive Medicine . . .' H. Frumkin: 'Beyond toxicity: Human health and the natural environment', American Journal of Preventive Medicine, volume 20, issue 3, 234–240

Page 85: 'A study in the Journal . . .' Woolery, A., Myers, H., Sternlieb, B., Zeltzer, L.: 'A yoga intervention for young adults with elevated symptoms of depression', Alternative Therapies in Health and Medicine, 10(2): 60–3 (Mar–Apr 2004).

Page 87: 'a recent Cochrane report . . .' Evans, J. G., Cochrane Review for Ginkgo Biloba for dementia and cognitive impairment, University of Oxford (2002).

Page 87: 'One study at the Oregon Health & Science University . . .' www.ohsu.edu.

Page 87: 'Another study published . . .' Nature Neuroscience, 10: 411–413 (2007).

Page 88: 'People who meditate every day . . .' Lazar, S. W., Kerr, C. E., et al: 'Meditation experience is associated with increased cortical thickness', NeuroReport, 16(17): 1893–1897 (28 November 2005).

Page 88: 'meditation can help regulate blood pressure . . .' Schneider, R. H., Alexander, C. N., et al: American Journal of Hypertension, 18(1): 88–98 (January 2005).

Chapter 7

Page 90: 'One government-funded study . . .' David Hide Asthma & Allergy Research Centre, St Mary's Hospital, Newport, Isle of Wight, 2000.

Page 90: 'Recent Durham . . .' Dr Madeleine Portwood www.durhamtrial.org.

Page 92: 'One study by the City University . . .' Taylor, T. S.: 'Children's Eyesight Study', published by Guide Dogs (December 2002).

Page 94: 'weight gain in the first year of college . . .' Morrow et al.: 'Freshman 15: Fact or Fiction?' Obesity, 14: 1438–1443 (2006).

Page 95: 'One study of the eating habits . . .' Haslam, W. J.: 'Obesity', The Lancet, volume 366, issue 9492, 1197–1209.

Page 95: 'Another study showed that newlyweds . . .' Professor Edward Abramson: To Have and To Hold, Kensington (1999).

Page 98: 'a study in the Lancet . . .' Lancet, 368: 261–262, 299–304 (2006).

Page 98: 'Bigger babies, better brains?' BMJ, 323(7314): 685 (22 September 2001).

Other publications

Patrick Holford: Optimum Nutrition for the Mind, Piatkus (2007).

Rita Carter: Mapping the Mind, Weidenfeld and Nicolson (2000).

Index